Single Session Therapy

Single Session Therapy: A Clinical Introduction to Principles and Practices explores the best ways to use a Single Session Therapy (SST) mindset to better achieve therapeutic goals.

This text presents comprehensive ideas and methods on how to make a single session of therapy efficient and effective with individuals, couples, and families, including those of various cultural backgrounds. It emphasizes productive mindsets and includes the following topics: concepts and methods, multi-theoretical approaches, training, various clinical problems and multicultural populations, the latest research findings, access, and implementation. Numerous clinical examples from different expert SST practitioners are presented and discussed throughout.

This book is an essential reference for professionals involved in brief therapy practice, research, and teaching.

Michael F. Hoyt, Ph.D., is a psychologist based in Mill Valley, California. He was one of the originators (with Moshe Talmon and Robert Rosenbaum) of the Single Session Therapy approach and is the author/coeditor of numerous publications on brief therapy, including *Brief Therapy and Beyond* (2017). He has been named a Distinguished Continuing Education Speaker by both the APA and the International Association of Marriage and Family Counselors, a Contributor of Note by the Milton H. Erickson Foundation, and was awarded the prestigious APF Cummings Psyche Prize for lifetime contributions to the role of psychologists in organized healthcare.

Single Session Therapy

A Clinical Introduction to Principles and Practices

MICHAEL F. HOYT

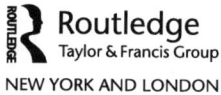

Routledge
Taylor & Francis Group

NEW YORK AND LONDON

First published 2025
by Routledge
605 Third Avenue, New York, NY 10158

and by Routledge
4 Park Square, Milton Park, Abingdon, Oxon, OX14 4RN

Routledge is an imprint of the Taylor & Francis Group, an informa business

ISBN: 978-1-032-74230-4 (hbk)
ISBN: 978-1-032-73689-1 (pbk)
ISBN: 978-1-003-46854-7 (ebk)

DOI: 10.4324/9781003468547

Typeset in Dante and Avenir
by codeMantra

To Judy Hoyt
Beloved Sister-in-Law

"The journey of a thousand miles begins with a single step."
  —Lao Tzu (6th century BCE)

"So teach us to number our days that we may get us a heart of wisdom."
  —Moses (*Psalms* 90: 12)

Contents

Preface

Single Session Therapy (SST) is therapy that is approached one-session-at-a-time. As my colleagues Jeff Young, Pam Rycroft, and I wrote in our editors' introduction to *Single Session Thinking and Practice in Global, Cultural, and Familial Contexts: Expanding Applications* (Hoyt, Young, & Rycroft, 2021, p. 3):

> The essence of single session thinking is to approach the first session as if it will be the only session, while creating opportunities for further work if it is requested by the client. What emerges is a collaborative, direct, and transparent approach to providing services that puts the client in a very active role in determining the focus and length of the work.

My "official" involvement with SST began sometime around 1986–1987 when two psychologist-colleagues, Moshe Talmon and Bob Rosenbaum, invited me to collaborate in a series of projects based on Moshe's discovery that one (1!) was actually the most common length of therapy for clients seen at the Hayward, California HMO clinic (Kaiser Permanente) where we were then working – regardless of whether the clients were seen by our Adult Team, Child and Family Team, or Chemical Dependency Team, and regardless of the particular therapist's identified theoretical orientation (psychodynamic, cognitive-behavioral, family systems, etc.).

As Moshe reported in the groundbreaking book *Single Session Therapy: Maximizing the Effect of the First (and Often Only) Therapeutic Encounter* (1990, pp. 6–10), he had been in the office of the Chief of Psychiatry looking at some computer printouts about department statistics when he noticed that ONE was the modal (most common) length of therapy across teams and providers. At first, he thought that this must mean that many patients had left unhappy (or "dropped out") after only one visit. But then he did an interesting and important thing: *he decided to contact the patients and see what actually had happened*. He called 200 patients. What he discovered was that most said that the one session was just what they had needed. They had achieved what they sought. In essence, they had "graduated," not "dropped out"!

After reviewing the literature and discovering a few scattered retrospective reports of unplanned one-session therapy successes, Moshe invited Bob Rosenbaum, and then me, to be research collaborators. We approached our employer, Kaiser Permanente, and proposed to do an investigation of possible planned one-session therapy. The affirmative findings of that study (and many others) are described in the chapters that follow.

Our first national presentations about SST occurred at the August 1987 American Psychological Association (APA) annual meeting in New York City, at the December 1988 Brief Therapy Conference (sponsored by the Milton H. Erickson Foundation) held in San Francisco, and at the August 1989 APA annual meeting in New Orleans. The resultant book, *Single Session Therapy: Maximizing the Effect of the First (and Often Only) Therapeutic Encounter* (Talmon, 1990), was the first prospective (and book-length) study of planned SST.

I say "official" involvement because, years earlier, my family and I had a personal experience in which we saw a therapist for one visit and what resulted was very helpful to us. I expect that most of us – as a therapist and/or as a client – may recall an experience of a successful one-session therapy – something good came of it, and there were no other meetings. Indeed, taking a moment to think about such experiences can help us to be open to the various possibilities of SST. Various friends, teachers, and entertainers, with a single remark, have at times also opened doors and helped me to shift my perspective and behavior. Additionally, I dabbled for years in Zen, Sufi, and Hasidic teaching tales (Paul Reps, Idries Shah, Martin Buber, et al.) in which someone awakens to wisdom as a result of a single encounter. Moreover, in my professional psychotherapy training, I had the good fortune to study with Carl Whitaker and with Bob and Mary Goulding, who frequently demonstrated the power of a single intervention. So, when Moshe and Bob asked me to join the SST project, I was primed.

In the subsequent years, I have had extensive clinical experience with SST (as well as other approaches, both short- and long-term) and have co-edited and co-authored several books on the topic (e.g., Hoyt & Talmon,

2014; Hoyt, Bobele, Slive, Young, & Talmon, 2018; Hoyt et al., 2021; and Hoyt & Cannistrà, 2023a; also see Talmon, Rosenbaum, Hoyt, & Short, 1990). This book goes well beyond those in that it presents, in one place, a multi-theoretical, multicultural approach with a mix of clinical models and many case examples as well as cautions to keep in mind. As will be apparent in the text and References, there are many colleagues who have also contributed good ideas. As one of the originators of the SST approach, I am pleased to offer my perspective, and hope that what follows will help professionals and graduate students to effectively and efficiently assist those who seek our help.

The Book in Hand

There are eight chapters (plus this Preface, Appendix A and Appendix B, References, and an Index). *Chapter 1: Introduction* discusses "What is SST?", highlights pro-SST attitudes, reviews the history of SST and its relationship to brief therapy, and describes the results of the first prospective SST clinical research study. *Chapter 2: The SST Mindset* addresses basic, underlying beliefs that guide SST, along with various "resistances." Drawing from several theories that can inform the practice of SST, a "Context of Competence" is discussed in which goals and resources meet via the therapeutic alliance. *Chapter 3: The Practice of SST* describes indications and contraindications as well as guideline steps. A "Temporal Structure" is presented to help organize tasks and useful questions, with special attention to how sessions begin and end. The options of by-appointment or walk-in meetings are also examined. *Chapter 4: SST Examples from the Literature – Methods and Models* and *Chapter 5: SST Examples from My Practice* provide numerous descriptions of SSTs with individuals, couples, and families. Brief quotations illustrate how different authors think of working in SST with various problems and allow readers to observe in action useful principles and effective language that can be adapted to readers' own clinical work. The cases involve a variety of theoretical orientations. Client details and circumstances have been changed throughout to protect confidentiality. Single-session thinking in humanitarian disaster situations, as well as the use of self-help SST, is also discussed. *Chapter 6: SST in Cross-Cultural Contexts* discusses the importance of cultural competence and gives various examples – some from the literature and some from my own practice. *Chapter 7: What Can We Learn from Our Internalized Clients?* offers an exercise to promote experiential learning opportunities. *Chapter 8: Summary, Additional Considerations, and Next Steps* reviews basics, discusses common errors in SST, and considers the importance of implementation and supervision, the use of single-session thinking in non-clinical situations, likely future trends, and take-aways and next steps. *Appendix A* provides an annotated sample of the quantitative evidence base, including studies of so-called "drop-outs" (who often actually have accomplished in one session what they wanted), that now supports SST. *Appendix B* provides checklists to help guide training exercises. All References are collected at the end, and an Index is provided.

Learning Objectives

Single Session Therapy: A Clinical Introduction to Principles and Practices is intended to help readers consider ways to embrace (when appropriate) an SST mindset and related methods in order to create possibilities for clients (and clinicians) to better use their competencies and resources to achieve therapeutic goals – maybe even in one planned-for session. Numerous examples from different expert SST practitioners are presented and discussed. This book is for clinicians interested in the possibility of a deliberate Single Session Therapy – although practitioners who do not plan for therapy to end after one session may also find much to consider. Many of the concepts and methods discussed herein (such as specific goal setting, building a therapeutic alliance, and ways to encourage clients' competencies) may help clinicians to be generally more effective and efficient, not just in SST.

Arnold Lazarus (1997, p. 6, italics in original) wrote: *"effective therapy depends far less on the hours you put in than on what you put into those hours."* Discussing the field of brief psychotherapy, he also kindly said: "Hoyt's *Brief Therapy and Managed Care* (1995) may be viewed as a standard reference and vade mecum [handbook or guide]." It is my hope that this volume (which does not discuss managed care) will update and exceed that tome. There is much here for practitioners of a wide variety of orientations to consider and use. As Federico Piccirilli and Lara Ermini (2021, p. 51) put it:

> But while certain epistemologies (such as radical constructivist or constructionist ones) or approaches (such as Ericksonian, humanistic, or systemic therapies) find it easier to adapt to typical SST ways of devising therapy, the fact we have trained colleagues with different orientations and approaches (cognitive-behavioral, strategic, psychodynamic, bioenergetic, Rogerian, narrative, etc.) and are ourselves trained in a 'mix' of styles (in terms of methodology and therapeutic approach)

demonstrates that anyone can understand and use the SST mindset for their own and their clients' benefit – without giving up their own preferences.

Although some new concepts and methods will be presented in what follows, I agreed when I read Brett Steenbarger (2012, p. 123, emphasis in original):

> My goal [...] is not to enable you to conduct brief therapy in the manner of recognized practitioners. I also do not intend to encourage you to do therapy my way. Instead, I wish you to *consider becoming more of the effective helper that you already are when you are at your best.* Identify what you are already doing when you are an efficient, effective facilitator of change, and then do those things more consistently and intentionally.

In introducing their particular SST approach, which they called Single-Session Experiential Therapy, Alvin Mahrer and Martine Roberge (1993, p. 180) extended "A Friendly Invitation to Try an Alternative Set of Cherished Truths about Psychotherapy":

> Almost every therapist has a personal package of cherished truths about psychotherapy. You have firmly entrenched beliefs about how to make sense of your patients, how change occurs, what is to change, and the directions of change that are worthwhile for each patient. Other approaches are seen through the perspective of your own cherished truths. If other approaches do not conform to or even violate your cherished truths, these other approaches are seen as alien, lesser, incomplete, and inadequate. [...] We offer you a friendly invitation to set aside your own cherished truths and to allow yourself to get inside another set of cherished truths. When you are done, you will go back to your own set of cherished truths, but of course we hope your ways of seeing how and what therapy can achieve will be enlarged a little.

Just as it is impossible for one book to teach completely an approach to therapy, there is no one "right" or "correct" way to do an SST (or any other therapy). My intention is to convey, as best I can, what I've learned over the past decades in the hope that you'll get what you need to begin doing intentional single session therapies with clients who want SST. Numerous examples from a range of theoretical orientations can be provided and general principles and guidelines can be offered and learned, but in the moment, it depends on the participants, their abilities and limitations, the situation, and everything else that may have an influence. Creativity involves "a genuine *process* of undetermined becoming: it cannot be the mere unfolding of an already completely determined sequence of steps to a ready-made conclusion" (Morson, 1994, p. 24, emphasis in original; also see Leslie, 2019). I like the way Nobel Prize laureate Bob Dylan (2022, p. 128) said it:

> One of the ways creativity works is the brain tries to fill in holes and gaps. We fill in missing bits of pictures, snatches of dialogue, we finish rhymes and invent stories to explain things we do not know.

Hillary and Brad Keeney (2013, p. 29) also encourage creating space for originality:

> The art of psychotherapy is found in the full complexity of its interactional choreography and cannot be reduced to an isolated action, expression, or prescription for behaving in a session […] So-called 'evidence-based' therapy research assumes the opposite. In the effort to produce standardized, 'best practice' models, therapy is reduced to particular isolated actions and sequences of actions to be replicated across multiple clinical situations. It follows that clients' problems must also be reduced to a set of isolated variables and lineal causal explanations in order to be 'treated' by the established model. The result is assembly line therapy that de-emphasizes creating skilled therapists who are able to work with the complexity of each unique client.

The book you have in hand, dear reader, is based on a workshop I have taught numerous times titled *SINGLE SESSION THERAPY* (see Hoyt, in press b). Sometimes the workshop's subtitle is *WHEN YOU HAVE A WHOLE HOUR*, borrowed from a chapter ("One Session at a Time: When You Have a Whole Hour") written by two esteemed colleagues, Monte Bobele and Arnie Slive (2014), who had earlier co-edited a book about SST with walk-in clients called *When One Hour is All You Have* (Slive & Bobele, 2011) and then realized the potential capaciousness of one session and recast the title. Sometimes the workshop's subtitle is *WHEN THE FIRST SESSION MAY BE THE LAST* (adapted from the subtitle of Talmon's [1990] book), and sometimes the workshop's subtitle is *MAKING THE MOST OF EACH SESSION* (emphasizing effectiveness and efficiency). They all highlight useful *PRINCIPLES AND PRACTICES*. Indeed, as we shall see, a LOT can get done in one meeting!

I have honed ideas based on much feedback of what audiences want and find useful. Various workshop handouts are adapted and included herein. I have endeavored to be both scholarly and personal, citing from the literature research and numerous clinical examples and also allowing my own voice to come through. Resonating with the observation of Rollo May, Ernest Angel, and Henri Ellenberger (1958, p. 8) that "human beings reveal themselves in art and literature and philosophy" and with Camille Paglia's (1992) call for a more widely integrated scholarship, in what follows I occasionally endeavor to adduce support and to "thicken description" (Geertz, 1973) with references to the broader humanities and popular culture. (Thank you, Will Shakespeare! Thank you, Bob Dylan!) I delight in finding connections and was pleased to read this passage in D.W. Winnicott's (1986, p. 120) *Home is Where We Start From*: "It is always a steadying thing to find that one's work links with entirely natural phenomena, and with the universals, and with what we expect to find in the best of poetry, philosophy and religion."[1]

I encourage readers to look for something new to learn – "look for the donut, not the hole" (a good single-session and brief therapy principle – look for what is there that can be used, not what is missing). Please be both receptive and generative, considering what is presented and finding ways to adapt and use some of it with your own style, cases, and situation. Apprehend more than is on the page. Were we in a workshop setting, I would also ask "What do you want to make sure we speak about?" and go to the board and write items. After exploring what would be indications that useful answers have been given, I would point out the process in which my inquiring about workshop attendees' goals parallels the process of attendee-therapists asking what goals their clients hope to achieve and how they'll know if they have achieved them. To emphasize the importance of having clear goals, I might also quip, using a metaphor from the world of golf (Hoyt, 2000), that "It's a long day on the course if you don't know where the hole is!" You might even pause now to think of (and maybe write down) a few questions that you hope we will address in what follows.

I don't have your specific questions, but it is intended that by the end of this book, readers will be able to:

---

1   For more extensive connecting of therapy with the broader humanities literature, see Hoyt (2017), especially Chapter 6 ("Some Stories Are Better than Others: A Postmodern Pastiche") and Chapter 15 ("Everyday Constructivism"). I agree with Sarah Bakewell (2023, p. 51): "Thus, to use language well [...] is about moving other people to emotion and recognition. It is a moral activity, because being able to communicate well is at the heart of *humanitas* – of being human in the fullest way."

1. List the basic features of brief therapy
2. Describe the tasks and skills, including useful questions and specific techniques, associated with different phases of each session (pre-early, middle, late, follow-through) and with overall treatment
3. Understand the single-session/one-at-a-time mindset
4. Analyze guidelines (indications, contraindications, steps) for SSTs
5. Apply single-session intervention strategies to some of their own clinical cases.

SST Can Help—But Does Not Solve Everything

Most of the time, SST can help with the psychological concerns of day-to-day life, assisting people to move forward, and can also be a valuable step in dealing with major challenges – but SST does not necessarily always produce dramatic shifts, major breakthroughs, or resolve life's dilemmas. As Talmon (1990, p. 111) reminds us, "Most of the successful SSTs we have studied do not resemble the demonstrations of master therapists in conferences or books." There are also problems (poverty, racism, sexism, ageism, militarism, homophobia, etc.) that may manifest psychologically but will ultimately require at least partial redress through sociopolitical means.

SST is therapy that is deliberately approached with the understanding that there may only be the one session. It is not therapy that was expected to go longer but ended before the therapist thought it should. Planned (by design, not default) SST is the topic of this book, although research (see Appendix A) has shown that many times clients who have been called "dropouts" actually got what they had sought in the one session. As we learned in the chart review of 200 unplanned cases who had not returned (see Talmon, 1990; discussed in Chapter 1), it can be instructive to call clients to see what happened and what might have made it better. Interest in planned SST, by appointment or by walk-in, is expanding rapidly, and this book is about what to do if your client wants and elects to attend only one session, not about what to do if your client doesn't come back.

SST (nor any therapy) does not always resolve problems, of course, but SST works for many people. Clients come at the moment of their choosing, when they are ready. SST is a *minimalist constructive approach* (Talmon, 2014, p. 31) in that it operates from the assumption that when clients feel encouraged and empowered, a small change often leads to larger ones – change "ripples" through the clients' internal and interpersonal systems. For many of us therapists, this has required shifting from being "The Expert" who "fixes" patients' problems to being more of a "privileged listener" who guides and facilitates clients' strengths and abilities to help them help themselves. One might say we move from being mechanics to gardeners (LeShan, 1982; Korngold, 2013, p. 164). As Talmon (2014, pp. 32–33) has written:

> Some people define SST and other ultra-brief therapies as a 'psychotically optimistic' way of conducting therapy. Trusting human potential, internal and external resources, as well as the ever-surprising capabilities of the mental immune system to recover and heal is indeed relentlessly optimistic. I agree and yet I tend to see SST more as a very realistic, practical, no bullshit, and down-to-earth form of therapy.

Therapy doesn't always have to be long term. At the same time, everything is not resolvable in a single session. People sometimes have terrible problems. Why doesn't everything just get fixed in one visit? And why do negative narratives persist? Sometimes it's brain stuff. Sometimes it's social situations. Sometimes it's habit. It's not a failure if it doesn't all get done in one session, but plenty of experiences have shown that in one session, especially if clinician and client are open to the possibility, a lot really can get done.

While SST (or other very brief therapy) doesn't solve all problems, by doing briefer therapy with some clients we will have more therapy resources available for those who truly need more therapy. (We also need more funding for mental-health services.) I see this as offering a choice and trying to "right size" the length of therapy rather than doing longer-than-necessary therapy with some clients. SST, however, should not be thought of as just or even primarily a strategy to conserve resources or manage waiting lists. More importantly, it's respectful and ethical to provide services that empower clients and help them to achieve their goals as soon as they can.

Acknowledgments

Many, many thanks:

- To the clients and patients, professors and students, authors and editors, and conference organizers and attendees who have taught me so much
- To my SST colleagues, especially my original Kaiser SST partners Moshe Talmon and Bob Rosenbaum, as well as Flavio Cannistrà, Jeff Young, Pam Rycroft, Arnie Slive, Monte Bobele, Windy Dryden, Martin Söderquist, Nancy McElheran, John Miller, Karen Young, Rubin Battino, and Jessica Schleider
- To Carl Whitaker and to Mary and Bob Goulding for their mentorship
- To other colleagues – including Steve Andreas, Pedro Vargas Avalos, Insoo Kim Berg, Simon Budman, Jon Carlson, Nick Cummings, Steve de Shazer, Edrick Dorian, Carol Erickson, Steven Friedman, John Frykman, Joe Goldfield, Eric Greenleaf, Alan Gurman, Jay Haley, Jürgen Hargens, Don Hidaldo, Richard Hill, Tobey Hiller, Chris Iveson, Murray Korngold, Jeffrey Kottler, Don Meichenbaum, Bill O'Hanlon, Clem Papazian, Harvey Ratner, Michele Ritterman, Ethan Schwartz, Dan Short, Terry Soo-Hoo, Grégoire Vitry, Michael White, and Phillip Ziegler – for many interesting discussions
- To The Bouverie Centre at La Trobe University in Melbourne, the Eastside Family Centre in Calgary, and the Italian Center for Single Session Therapy in Rome for organizing and hosting excellent international SST symposia

- To Kaiser Permanente and the Stanley Garfield Award for Clinical Innovation, who granted time for the original Talmon-Rosenbaum-Hoyt SST project
- To the APF Cummings Psyche Prize for its generous support of my writing
- To Sarah Rae and Routledge Publishers for embracing this project, to Pragati Sharma for her editorial attention to a myriad of details, and to Uma Maheswari and CodeMantra for its excellent production
- To the Mill Valley Public Library for continued reference assistance
- To Darrell Coughlan for IT support
- To LexiLou (and Kingster, too) for being themselves
- To my dear wife Jennifer, for endless love, friendship, our home, and for her forbearance and good counsel.

Introduction: What Is SST?

1

Single Session Therapy (SST) is therapy that is understood, from the beginning, to likely comprise a single session. Since the publication of *Single Session Therapy: Maximizing the Effect of the First (and Often Only) Therapeutic Encounter* (Talmon, 1990), there has been abundant research (some highlighted below and more in Appendix A) showing that many clients may not return for further meetings – and that the first (and only) session is all they want and need. Actually, ZERO is the most common length of treatment: people think they should go to therapy, but never do! Amongst those who actually attend, studies repeatedly indicate that one session is the most common length of treatment, followed by two, then three. While some clients will sooner or later return for another session or sessions, the fact that many people only attend one session is a prime reason, as the subtitle of Talmon's innovative 1990 book put it, to study and develop ways for "maximizing the effect of the first (and often only) therapeutic encounter."

Talmon (1990 p. xvi) wrote:

> *Single-Session Therapy* shows how to use single sessions to prompt substantial changes in patients' lives. It explains how to capitalize on it, plan for it, and change normal therapeutic practices in order to support more creativity as well as effectiveness; it provides guidance on how to use time differently, how to foster readiness and motivation, and how to combine the necessary intake-diagnostic process with that of promoting change.

DOI: 10.4324/9781003468547-1

That is the subject of this book.

SST is a planned, deliberate approach to "capture the moment" (Young & Rycroft, 1997; Hoyt & Talmon, 2014), to make the most of the first session. As Hymmen, Stalker, and Cait (2013, p. 61) put it:

> SST refers to a conscious approach to make the most of the first session knowing it may be the only session the client decides to attend – not to the situation where there is an expectation that the client will attend multiple sessions but chooses to attend just one.

SST is not a particular psychotherapy theoretical orientation (such as psychodynamic, cognitive-behavioral, and solution-focused). Talmon (2014, p. 31) explained:

> When we started our SST project, Rosenbaum had trained in brief psychodynamic therapy and was then fascinated with non-directive hypnosis à la Milton Erickson. Hoyt had done an internship with Carl Whitaker, trained in brief psychodynamic therapy, and was then taken by the work of Mary and Bob Goulding (1979), which combined Transactional Analysis (TA) and Gestalt into what they called Redecision Therapy, a very directive form of treatment. I was primarily a systemic therapist working with the Child and Family Team while Hoyt and Rosenbaum worked with the Adult Team. When we started the project I was quite intrigued by the simple elegance of solution-focused therapy developed by de Shazer, Berg, et al. (de Shazer, 1985, 1988) in Milwaukee. I met them shortly before our project started and they were a main force in spreading the word about our initial findings long before we published anything.

SST is at heart an approach to service delivery. Jeff Young (2018, p. 44) writes:

> [A] fundamental definition of Single Session Therapy could be everything that derives attitudinally, clinically, and organizationally from accepting three findings, two backed by research and the third by our clinical experience. Finding #1: that the most common number of service contacts that clients attend is one, followed by two, followed by three… irrespective of diagnosis, complexity, or the severity of their problem (Talmon, 1990). Finding #2: that the majority (often above 70–80%) of those people who attend only one session, across a range of therapies, report that the single session was adequate given their

current circumstance (Talmon, 1990; Bloom, 2001; Campbell, 2012). Finding #3: possibly the hardest finding to accept, is that it seems impossible to accurately predict who will attend only one session and who will attend more, a proposition that has significant clinical and organizational ramifications.

The essence of SST (and by extension, single session thinking and practice) is to approach each session with the idea that it may be the only session. *SST is therapy that the therapist and client expect, from the beginning, to be a single visit.* As Flavio Cannistrà (2018/2021a, p. 119) has put it: "SST's advantage is that it can be applied in different contexts and by different practitioners, regardless of orientation. The aim, in fact, is always to maximize the effectiveness of every single – often the only – encounter."

SST typically involves the "50-minute hour," a standard office session, which is usually adequate; but particularly with a couple or family, a 60–90-minute SST session may be helpful to allow for a complete process or intervention. In Chapter 3, we'll discuss options regarding scheduling longer and shorter sessions.

If it takes more than one session, it doesn't mean it was a "single session failure" – it just means it took more than one session. As I like to say at the beginning of a workshop,

> I don't believe in brief or single session therapy, and I also don't believe in long-term therapy. What I believe in and advocate for is appropriate, clinically sound, help-the-client-make-a-change-as-soon-as-possible therapy and try to avoid the argument of how brief is brief and how long is long. There are people I've seen for 20 or more sessions, and it was time sensitive, time efficient, brief, meaning given their internal and external challenges and resources, every moment was needed; and there are other people I've seen for two sessions and it was at least twice as long as it should have been. The goal is being effective and efficient, no more than needed, making the most of each session.

The idea of a single session of therapy potentially being sufficient concentrates the mind, helps to structure the meeting, and encourages hope and effort. As we will see in the chapters ahead, there is a lot of clinical experience and research evidence to support the practice of SST.

Here is a list of pro-SST attitudes (from Hoyt et al., 1992, pp. 61–62) that will help set the stage for subsequent discussions.

- View each session as a whole, potentially complete in itself. Expect change.
- The power is in the patient. Never underestimate your client's strength.
- This is it. All you really have is now.
- The therapeutic process starts before the first session and will continue long after it.
- The natural process of life is the main force of change.
- You don't have to know everything in order to be effective.
- You don't have to rush or reinvent the wheel.
- More is not necessarily better. *Better* is better. A small step can make a big difference.
- Helping people as quickly as possible is practical and ethical. It will encourage patients to return for help if they have other problems and will also allow therapists to spend more time with patients who require longer treatments.

Single session therapists employ a variety of theoretical models and work in diverse settings including clinics, private practice offices, hospitals, "second-opinion" consultations, and clinical demonstration interviews. What these practices all have in common is the idea that *all we really have is now and this one meeting may be enough – or may be all that the client will decide to attend.* When therapy is organized with a planned and deliberate attitude that one session may be sufficient, clients frequently decide one session is adequate and choose to attend only that one session; and most report satisfaction and benefit.

SST is not a panacea and should not be oversold, imposed, or forced (see Cummings, 2000). As Windy Dryden (2019b, p. 16) has written, "SST should not be foisted on reluctant therapists, nor on reluctant clients. It is best practiced when clients see the potential in it, and therapists embrace the challenge of helping clients in the shortest possible period." When offered as a choice, many people choose one session and find it helpful. SST is responsive to the pattern of many clients' natural help-seeking behavior. It is respectful and collaborative, with the client determining the focus and length of therapy. Sometimes in one session a problem is "solved" or "resolved" – other times things just get "unstuck" and "processed" and maybe coped with or managed better. A client may use a single session to make a significant life change, or to take a step in the right direction; or as a "sounding board" to consider options, and/or validate their thoughts and efforts; or perhaps to gain support and avoid a worsening of symptoms. As Bob Rosenbaum (2021) notes, change can occur both gradually and suddenly. The basic idea is to make the most of each session and to proceed as though the session may be the last. Each session is bespoke: one size does not fit all.

Single Session Therapy/One-at-a-Time (SST/OAAT): What's in a Name?

The term *Single Session Therapy* (SST) indicates that there will be one meeting to provide psychological services:

> *single* – each meeting is seen as an episode complete unto itself, a 'stand-alone unity' (James, 2014, p. xiv), having a beginning, middle, and end. It's a planned, deliberate one-time event although another single session (or sessions) could occur later
>
> *session* – a meeting or gathering (encounter). This could be in person, on the telephone, or online
>
> *therapy* – 'Time-sensitive treatment to relieve psychological distress and/or promote growth' or 'The development of a collaborative alliance and an emphasis on patient/client strengths in the service of an efficient attainment of co-created goals.'
>
> (from Hoyt, 2009a)

As Jeff Young (2018) has written, the name *Single Session Therapy* is deliberately disruptive. It is "in your face," the word *single* challenging assumptions that therapy must be a prolonged process.[1]

Another, less provocative but closely related term is *One at a Time* (OAAT; Hoyt, 2011), which also emphasizes the idea that therapy is approached *one session at a time* (Slive & Bobele, 2011; Bobele & Slive, 2014). It is important to recognize that "One at a Time" doesn't necessarily mean "only one time." Another session (or sessions) could occur later. An additional oft-heard term is *walk-in*, designating those who arrive without prior appointment, but to my ear, it doesn't make clear by itself the single session/one-at-a-time aspect. I prefer *walk-in SST* (or *"SST by walk-in"*) to highlight that it's a single session unto itself, rather than just walking in to start ongoing therapy. Other variants like *single session thinking and practice, single session intervention, single session consultation*, and *single session work* have their place and carry various implications, but I like "SST": it's clear, provocative, and consistent with the literature.[2]

---

1   Although SST is first and foremost a way to provide services that empower clients to achieve their goals as soon as they can, and not simply a cost-saving strategy, the titles of Carol Shaw Austad's 1996 book, *Is Long-Term Psychotherapy Unethical? Toward a Social Ethic in an Era of Managed Care;* and Steven Friedman's (1997) book, *Time-Effective Psychotherapy: Maximizing Outcomes in an Era of Minimized Resources*, both point toward the practical value of focused, goal-oriented therapy.

2   Talmon (2014, p. 30) reports: " I first titled my [1990] book *Once Upon a Therapy* to hint at the possibility of being seen only once but mostly to indicate my realization that therapy is different

We all don't do the same thing under the heading *SST* – and don't have to. As we will see, some SST practitioners are more CBT, some more SFBT, some more narrative, some more Ericksonian, some more strategic problem-solving, some more multi-theoretical/eclectic, etc. For an extended discussion of SST terminology, including non-English language variants, see Hoyt, Young, and Rycroft (2021, pp. 11–15).

SST also is not *crisis intervention* (unless crisis intervention turns out to be what is called for once the session begins – Hoyt & Talmon, 2014; Bobele & Slive, 2015; for a couple of examples of using SST principles in humanitarian crisis situations, see Chapter 6 this volume.). Generally speaking, crisis intervention involves short-term, first-aid techniques to stabilize a situation and minimize and prevent permanent damage. By contrast, SST is non-emergency planned-to-be-one-session therapy, by appointment or by walk-in. More about ways to offer access to SST will be discussed in Chapter 3.

The terms *patient* and *client* each carry certain implications (see Hoyt, 1979, 1985/2017, pp. 1–5 and 217–218). The Kaiser study (Talmon, 1990) was conducted within the context of a medical healthcare organization, so the term *patient* was used. *Client* tends to emphasize a more egalitarian and less hierarchical therapeutic relationship with a subsequent de-emphasis on implications of pathology, diagnosis, and expert (top-down) treatments in favor of more collaborative/strengths-based approaches (see Hoyt, 1994a, pp. 2–4). Paralleling the question of what to call the recipient of services is the question of what to call the person(s) offering those services – *therapist, counselor, provider, practitioner*, etc. As noted in Hoyt and Talmon (2014, p. 11):

> What one calls the participants and the process (*therapy? counseling? treatment? intervention? consultation? facilitation? work? practice? meeting? encounter? conversation? coaching?*) helps to establish a meaning context (topics, roles, power relations, ideas about how change occurs) and thus influences their work together.

---

than what I assumed, expected, or had been told in my training" – but his editor "insisted that *Single Session Therapy* is clearer and more 'catchy' and we compromised by adding the excellent but somewhat long subtitle: *Maximizing the Effect of the First (and Often Only) Session*." L.-G. Öst (e.g., Öst et al., 2001; also Ollendick & Davis, 2013) has offered the acronymic term *OST* (!) for *One Session Treatment*. Rosenbaum (2008) considered calling it "moment-by-moment therapy." Bennett, Myles-Hooton, Schleider & Shafran (2022) refer to "brief and low intensity interventions" and Schleider (2024) refers to "little treatments, big effects" and "meaningful moments" and, as discussed in Chapter 2, prefers the more generic term *Single Session Intervention* to include digital, self-administered programs that do not involve a trained therapist.

However, the client arrives – by appointment or walk-in (or telephone call-in or online click-in) – once they arrive, there are essentially three ways one could have an SST:

1. The client/patient stops unilaterally even though the therapist thinks therapy should continue. This is often called "dropout," although considerable research (see Appendix A) has shown that people who stop after one session, even if it was not predetermined SST, have often achieved what they sought and are thus actually "completers" or "graduates" rather than "drop-outs";

2. The therapist stops unilaterally even though the client wants to continue. In reality, this only happens if the client is unable to pay the therapist's fee or the client is so difficult or unpleasant that regardless of ability to pay the therapist does not want to have additional meetings; or

3. The client and therapist agree to one session and at the end of the meeting mutually agree that the one session was enough – at least for now. (Remember: "One-at-a-Time" doesn't necessarily mean "Only-One-Time.")

I'm in favor of the third, of course. Insistence produces resistance, imposition produces opposition, and push produces pushback – so invitation (not insistence or imposition) is the key. Saying "Would you be interested ..." is more likely to gain productive cooperation than "You only get..."

Relationship of SST to Brief Therapy

SST is defined by its intention to provide a complete therapeutic experience (beginning, middle, end) in one meeting. More generally, brief therapy (which may draw from different theoretical orientations, as does SST) is characterized by its intention to be concise, not necessarily one session but "not one more session than necessary" (de Shazer, 1991a, p. ix). When I asked Jay Haley (personal communication, December 1995) why they had named it "Brief Therapy," he explained that it was simply "to clearly say that it was not long-term therapy, which was primarily psychoanalytic back then." Brief therapy is more open-ended, or at least not so delimited. Brevity does not necessarily mean superficial; the right haiku can be much more to the point and soul stirring than a long, plodding novel – or therapy (Hoyt, 2014, p. 68).

The term "Brief Therapy" has sometimes been used to refer to a tradition based specifically on a social constructionist (Gergen & McNamee, 1991) and radical constructivist (Watzlawick, 1984; von Glaserfeld, 1995) theoretical throughline featuring Ericksonian, MRI, and solution-focused contributions – but the term can also be used more generically to include approaches informed by psychodynamic, cognitive-behavioral, and other concepts. Brief therapy is not planned SST, but the two significantly overlap in their focus on goal-directed efficiency.

Cutting across different "schools" or theoretical orientations, here are the basic features of brief therapy (see Budman, Hoyt, & Friedman, 1992; Hoyt, 1995a, 2009c, 2017):

- *Rapid and positive alliance.* "Common factors" research (Duncan, Miller, Wampold, & Hubble, 2009) shows a positive therapeutic alliance to be a strong predictor of a good therapy outcome. The connection is important: clients usually won't care what you know until they know that you care. The alliance begins in the client's mind when they think about having an appointment. Our expectations and mindset also prefigure (see Chapter 2) our "theory countertransference" (Hubble & O'Hanlon, 1992) as seen in statements such as "They've been in the hospital – this is going to take a long time" and "Damn – she's a borderline." Sometimes it is better to think of our responses more positively, as "client-inspired therapist contributions" (Hoyt, 2017, pp. 179–188). Are you hosting a therapeutic conversation? (Furman & Ahola, 1992). If you meet in the waiting room, do you say their name and maybe shake their hand? Do you walk side-by-side to your office, or do they follow behind you?
- *Goal focus.* A golf flag could be here to remind us that "It's a long day on the course if you don't know where the hole is" (Hoyt, 1996a/2017, p. 33). Every stroke should be purposeful – why are we talking about this rather than that? What intention or logic underlies a therapist's actions – what result does the therapist expect from a particular action? Both *why* (purpose) and *how* (method, skillfulness) are important. A technique in different situations could serve different purposes (e.g., to build alliance, to establish a goal, to block an unsuccessful attempted solution, to identify a strength, etc.) – see Cannistrà (2019) and Cannistrà and Hoyt (2020/2023).

  As Jay Haley (1977, p. 9) put it, "If therapy is to end properly, it must begin properly – by negotiating a solvable problem." To move "from problem to solution" (George, Iveson, & Ratner, 1990), it will help to get specifics of what the client(s) will be doing differently when the presenting problem is no longer present. Vague complaints such as "low self-esteem," "poor communication," and "unhappy" are "suitcase words" (Ziegler & Hoyt, 2023) that need to be unpacked: "Self-esteem" is how one rates or esteems oneself, so what will the person be thinking differently about themselves when therapy is effective? How will they be communicating – what will they be saying differently, with whom? What will be some signs that they are moving toward "positive self-esteem," "good communication," and "happy"? Vague goals make for vague therapy (see Eisenthal & Lazare, 1976a, 1976b; Dattilio, 1998). de Shazer (1991b, p. 112) describes the general characteristics of well-formed goals: they are small rather than large; salient to clients; articulated in specific, concrete behavioral terms; achievable within the practical contexts of clients' lives; perceived by clients as involving their own hard work; seen as the "start of something" and not just as the "end of something"; and treated as involving new behavior rather than the absence or cessation of existing behavior (e.g., falling asleep rather than stopping insomnia, communicating calmly rather than arguing).[3] What would that look like? "If the man or the woman on the moon looked through the window, what would he see or she see you doing differently?" Get the description to a size where it's achievable. A lot of the SST mindset is looking in detail for where the client wants to go – and then how they can get there.

- *Clear definition of client/therapist responsibilities/activities.* What is our role as therapist, and what is the client/patient's role? We should not be authoritarian, but there are times we can serve as authorities – we may have ideas and information that would be useful to the client. Some therapy may take place in the office, but the client can be charged with responsibility to do homework (which may be called *practice opportunities* or *learning moments* if the term "homework" is off-putting – discussed further in Chapter 3). The passive "When I feel better I'll do it" can sometimes be productively met with "Actually, it's when you do it that you'll feel better." This is a form of what CBT therapists (see Jacobson, Martell, & Dimidgian, 2001; Read, Mazzucchelli, & Kane, 2016) might call *behavior activation* – getting clients involved in activities that have the potential for positive reinforcements to improve their mood.
- *Emphasis on strengths/competencies, with an expectation of change producing hope* (see Battino, 2006, 2014; Hoyt, 2021). We may speak suppositionally ("*When* things are better …" rather than "*If* things get better"). The Miracle Question (de Shazer, 1988) asks "Suppose tonight there is a miracle. When you awake tomorrow morning, what will be the first thing you'll notice that tells you the problem is gone? And then what?" Other questions similar to de Shazer's Miracle Question include Alfred Adler's (1964) "What would change if we waved a magic wand and all your problems were solved?" and Milton Erickson's (1954a) Crystal Ball

---

3   These are similar to (but somewhat different from) the concrete and positive terms that Doran (1981) refers to as S.M.A.R.T. goals: Specific, Measurable, Attainable, Realistic, and Time-bound.

Technique: "Imagine a time in the future when the problems are gone. What would that look like? Describe the steps you took to get there." As Bobele, López, Scamardo, and Solórzano (2008, p. 87) put it:

> Our single-session model normalizes the client's experience as much as possible. Change was promoted by emphasizing strengths, abilities, and skills. [...] The therapist must be willing to approach clients from the stance, 'Each session has the potential of being a single-session,' to create an expectancy of change.

• *Novelty – changing "the viewing and doing"* (O'Hanlon & Wilk, 1987; O'Hanlon & Weiner-Davis, 1989; O'Hanlon, 1990). More of the same does not make a change. The need for something new sometimes can be inspired by quoting the adage, "If you don't change directions, you'll wind up where you're heading"; or by asking the motivational question T.V.'s Dr. Phil sometimes asks: "How's that workin' for you?" (If it was "workin'" they wouldn't be sitting on his studio couch crying their eyes out, would they?)[4] William James (1890) said "A difference which makes no difference is no difference at all," Gregory Bateson (1979, p. 92) said that "Information is news of a difference," Steve de Shazer suggested "putting difference to work," and Bill O'Hanlon (1999) advised "do one thing different."

As Watzlawick, Weakland, and Fisch (1974, p. 95) wrote:

> To reframe [...] means to change the conceptual and/or emotional setting or viewpoint in relation to which a situation is experienced and to place it in another frame which fits the 'facts' of the same concrete situation equally well or even better, and thereby changes its entire meaning.[5]

---

4 Some other statements that highlight the problem-generating cost of rigid avoidance and the necessity of change can be seen in this therapist statement from Nardone and Salvini (2007/2018, p. 24): "Well, what we have said so far brought to my mind a phrase by a well-known poet, Fernando Pessoa, who wrote, 'You bear the wounds of the battles you never fought', and I would add – the wounds of evaded battles never truly heal." Shakespeare's lines in *Julius Caesar* (Act II, Scene 2), "A coward dies a thousand times before his death, the valiant taste of death but once" also suggest the high cost of excessive avoidance. If I were talking with an avid golfer (see Hoyt, 1996a), I might say: "You know, the more you try to avoid the water by overcorrecting, the worse your slice will get – you'll need to face the hazard to get around it." What is important is that the metaphor makes emotional sense to the client.

5 Another expression – perhaps Richer, more inviting, more redolent with possibilities – comes from Walt Whitman's *Leaves of Grass* (1881–1892/1940, Stanza 21):

> I am the poet of the Body and I am the poet of the Soul,
> The pleasures of heaven are with me and the pains of hell are with me,
> The first I graft and increase upon myself,
> The latter I translate into a new tongue.

de Shazer (1988, p. 103) notes: "when the therapist frames things differently and responds differently from what the client expects, the client will then come to see himself differently. Thus the client's frame may be placed in doubt and more useful behavior might follow."

"Difference" can be introduced with explanation, education, reframing, metaphor, a well-timed psychodynamic transference interpretation, appropriate therapist self-disclosure ("My son is in college now, but my wife and I felt that way the first time we went out after he was born"), identifying exceptions to the problem. With one step – the right step – clients can do something different to break out of their painful, reiterating traps. As James Gustafson (2005, p. xiii, italics in original) noted,

> very brief psychotherapy is about *the moment of change being only a single step* which is unprecedented, as in the 'new beginning' of Michael Balint (1968), or a single step which has been taken before but is not allowed to slip away.

Michele Ritterman (2009, pp. 129–130) reminds us that a train, taking just a slight angle onto a different track, can wind up in a brand new place. As Malcom Gladwell (2000) has written, little things can make a big difference.

- *Here-and-now (and <u>next</u>) orientation.* Brief therapists sometimes "take history" to join with the client and to better understand what they have experienced as well as to "make history" by looking for overlooked exceptions and strengths (Hoyt, 2017, pp. 95–105). It's okay to occasionally glance in the rear-view mirror, but if you want to go forward, as Milton Erickson (1954b, p. 127) reminded us, "Emphasis should be placed more upon what the patient does in the present and will do in the future than upon a mere understanding of why some long-past event occurred."

- *Time sensitivity/intermittency.* Some now, some later: Clients may come in to get help getting "unstuck" but will not need us to then go on the journey of life with them. Therapy may be *intermittent* (Cummings & Sayama, 1995), provided at the *point of need* (Dryden, 2019a). If your car gets stuck by the roadside, the AAA person may come out and help you to get going again, or may even tow you into the shop if you need a bigger repair; but it would be weird, would it not, if after you got going, he/she said: "Now I want you to come by the shop every week for the next year so I can keep an eye on things."

In "How I Embody a Narrative Constructive Approach," I emphasized (2002, p. 288) the importance of noticing your noticing, paying attention to the way that you choose where to place your attention, and concluded with the hope "that you will allow for the growth of more stories that bring you more of what you want. We all get to decide: *Will our life be prose, or poetry?*" Sometimes this can happen in a single session!

The History and Research Evidence for SST

Sigmund Freud, often thought of as the father of psychoanalysis and long-term therapy, was also the first to report successful SSTs. In one case, he met with an emotionally upset young woman named Katharina (her parents were the innkeepers where Freud and his family were on vacation in the Alps), and in another, he met with the famous music composer Gustav Mahler (who was having sexual and marital problems). We don't know exactly what they talked about, but we do know that they knew they would only be meeting one time – and from reports (Breuer & Freud, 1893–1895/1955, Case 4; Kuehn, 1965), we know that the one-session therapies with Katharina and with Mahler were successful. In another instance (see https://www.telegraph.co.uk/news/worldnews/ europe/austria/1517214/Freuds-last-patient-recalls meeting-that-saved-my-life. html; Slavin & Rahmani, 2016), Freud met with an adolescent young woman. Seventy years later, she said "Those 45 minutes changed my life." Many of the cases of the famous psychiatrist-hypnotherapist Milton Erickson were also one session long, a single session actually being his most common length of treatment (Hoyt, 2000c) – Erickson is discussed more in Chapter 4.

Throughout the years, scattered reports about successful single sessions have appeared in the professional psychotherapy literature (see Sproel, 1975; Bloom, 1981/1995; Rockwell & Pinkerton, 1982; Campbell, 1999; Hurn, 2005; Cameron, 2007; O'Neill, 2017). Here are a few:

- Lewis Wolberg (1965, p. 138), who edited the first book in the U.S. about brief therapy: "Human warmth and feelings, experienced by a patient in one session with an empathic therapist, may achieve more profound alterations than years with a probing, detached therapist intent on wearing out resistance."
- D.W. Winnicott (1958, p. 261), child psychoanalyst: "The idea behind playing as communication is that if we know about regression in the analytic hour, we can meet it immediately and in this way enable certain patients [...] to make the necessary regressions in short phases, perhaps even almost momentarily."
- K.K. Lewin (1970, pp. 49–69): "If a patient is seen for even a single interview, it should be a therapeutic experience. Sometimes it is not enough to offer the patient a mirror in which to see himself; often he must be encouraged to open his eyes and be shown where to look. [... The] interview becomes an awakening, an intense stimulation of mind and spirit, and hopefully a corrective emotional experience."

- Arnold Lazarus (1971, p. 50), the originator of multimodal therapy: "In a surprising number of cases, people may require no more than an initial interview to precipitate lasting change and achieve profound behavioral readjustment."
- Eric Berne (quoted in Goulding & Goulding, 1979, p. 4), the originator of Transactional Analysis: "Before each group session I pause and ask myself, 'How can I cure everyone in this room today?'"
- David Malan and his psychodynamically oriented associates at the Tavistock Clinic in London reported encouraging research results and wrote (Malan, Health, Bacal, & Balfour, 1975, p. 126): "Clearly psychiatrists who undertake consultations should not automatically assign patients to long-term psychotherapy or even to brief therapy but should be aware of the possibility that a single dynamic interview may be all that is needed."[6]
- Bill O'Hanlon and Michele Weiner-Davis (1989, p. 77–78), developers of solution-oriented therapy, similarly opined: "We have observed enough 'one-session cures' to be utterly convinced that they are neither flukes, miracles, nor magic. Rather, something powerfully therapeutic occurs in the interaction between therapist and client during these sessions."
- Carl Whitaker (1990/1992, p. 18), originator of symbolic-experiential family therapy and Evolution of Psychotherapy Conference faculty member: "I've always thought that my most successful cases were those that lasted only one session. The family came together, something powerful happened that compelled them to make changes. Longer therapies meant that it took longer to reach this 'critical mass' or that we were missing some important aspect."
- Ellen Quick (1996, p. 166), developer of a strategic solution-focused approach to brief therapy: "On some occasions the client is satisfied with a single session and does not need to reschedule at all. [...] The therapy is brief, not because of benefit [insurance] limitations, but because what is needed for now has been completed."

---

6 *As recounted in Hoyt (2017, p. 11), I am reminded of an experience I had long ago when I visited the Short-Term Therapy Seminar at the renowned Tavistock Clinic (Malan, 1976a, 1976b) in London. Cases were presented and I was asked to comment, which I did with some trepidation. We got into a discussion about length of treatment. I indicated that at the clinic where I was then working we generally saw patients for twelve sessions, a number that followed Mann's (1973) time-limited psychotherapy model and allowed for a good research design (Horowitz et al., 1984). "Here at the Tavistock we allow trainees thirty-five to forty sessions. It allows for wasting time and making mistakes," I was told. "Well, in America we're more efficient," I responded. "We find that we can waste time and make mistakes in twelve sessions!" waste time and make mistakes in twelve sessions!"

- The July 2018 issue of *O: The Oprah Magazine* (with a monthly circulation of 2.5 million) had a cover story called "Bull's Eye! One-and-Done Sessions Give New Meaning to the Phrase *Targeted Therapy*" (DeMelo, 2018).
- David Burns (2020, p. 34): "In contrast to *Feeling Good* (Burns, 1980), which was all about the cognitive revolution, this book [*Feeling Great*] is about the motivation revolution. It is based on the simple idea that we sometimes get 'stuck' in depression and anxiety because we have mixed feelings about recovery [...] Through a new approach called TEAM-CBT, you can overcome this resistance and achieve recovery quickly [p. xv] [...] You *can* change the way you feel, and it *can* happen really fast."

As mentioned earlier, my own involvement with SST began in the mid-1980s, when I joined with Moshe Talmon and Bob Rosenbaum in the prospective research project we did at the Kaiser Permanente Medical Center in Hayward, California. Although we were influenced by solution-focused, psychodynamic, cognitive-behavioral, redecision, structural family therapy, symbolic-experiential therapy, and strategic Ericksonian approaches, we did not employ one model of therapy but used whatever skills the therapist and client could apply. We saw 58 consecutive outpatients,[7] ages 8–80 with a wide variety of diagnoses, and found (see Talmon, 1990):

- Over half of the patients (58.6%) elected to complete their therapy in one session even when more sessions were available;
- More than 88% reported significant improvement in their original "presenting complaint" and more than 65% also reported "ripple" improvements in related areas of functioning; and
- While not experimentally assigned to one session or longer, on follow-up, there was no difference in satisfaction and outcome scores between those who chose to stop after one visit (SST) versus those who continued for more sessions.

In the early 1990s, walk-in single session services were developed at the Eastside Family Centre in Calgary, Canada (see Slive, MacLaurin, Oaklander, & Amundson, 1995; Miller & Slive, 2004; Stewart et al., 2018; McElheran, 2021); there were concomitant developments at the Reach Out Centre for Kids (ROCK) in the province of Ontario, Canada, and there are now dozens of walk-in SST clinics in Ontario (Young, 2018). Walk-in SSTs were taken by

---

7   Actually, 60 cases were seen (20 by each co-investigator), but two subsequently moved out-of-state and so calculations are based on the 58 for which follow-up data were available.

Monte Bobele to Our Lady of the Lake University in San Antonio, Texas, where they are taught to graduate students and provided to the community (see Slive & Bobele, 2011). Important SST work was (and is) also being done at The Bouverie Centre of La Trobe University in Melbourne, Australia (Young, Rycroft, & Weir, 2014; Rycroft & Young, 2021). In a large-scale study in Australia (Weir, Wills, Young, & Perlesz, 2008), involving more than 100,000 consumers, 42% chose to have one session even when more sessions were readily available. Moshe Talmon in Israel; Bob Rosenbaum in California; Arnie Slive and Monte Bobele (2011) in Texas; Windy Dryden in England (2017, 2019a, 2019b); Martin Söderquist (2018, 2021, 2023) and Lars-Göran Öst et al. (see Ollendick & Davis, 2013) in Sweden; John Miller (2014; Miller, Xing, Yaorui, & Yilin, 2021) in China and in Cambodia (Miller, Platt, & Conroy, 2018); Karen Young (2018) and Nancy McElheran (2021) in Canada; Jessica Schleider and associates (Bennett et al., 2022; Schleider, 2024) in the U.S.; and Flavio Cannistrà and Federico Piccirilli (2018/2021a, 2021b) in Italy (plus others) have all made and continue to make important contributions. (For additional SST history, see Talmon, 1990; Slive & Bobele, 2011; Hoyt and Talmon, 2014; Hoyt, Bobele, Slive, Young, & Talmon, 2018a; Hoyt et al., 2021; Cannistrà & Piccirilli, 2018/2021a; Dryden 2017, 2019a, 2019b; Söderquist, 2023.)

There also have been four international SST symposia, each resulting in a coedited book:

a.   In March 2012 on Phillip Island (near Melbourne, Australia) – see Hoyt and Talmon (2014)
b.   In September 2015 in Banff, Canada – see Hoyt et al. (2018a)
c.   In October 2019 in Melbourne – see Hoyt et al., (2021)
d.   In November 2023 in Rome, Italy – see Cannistrà and Hoyt (in press).

Reflecting the expanding international interest in SST, in addition to the English-language editions of these symposia books, a version of Hoyt and Talmon (2014) is available in Italian; a version of Hoyt et al. (2018) in Spanish; and a combination of selected chapters from Hoyt et al. (2018) and Hoyt et al. (2021) has appeared in German. A Spanish version of Slive and Bobele (2011) and a Swedish version of Söderquist (2023) are available. There is a book about SST in Dutch by Helen van Empel (in press), Talmon's original 1990 *Single Session Therapy* has also appeared in many world languages.

An annotated list of research studies, illustrating that SST/OAAT is frequent and effective in a variety of settings with a range of problems, is provided in Appendix A. Numerous clinical examples will be presented and discussed in Chapters 4–6, but first let us consider in Chapters 2 and 3 the SST mindset and some ways it gets translated into practice.

The SST Mindset   **2**

Mindset refers to the set of basic beliefs and attitudes that influence how one thinks, feels, and behaves in any given situation (Hoyt & Cannistrà, 2023a). To my mind (see Hoyt, 2023), while an assortment of theoretical orientations has been shown to be useful, underlying SST are four fundamental ("mindset") ideas:

1. Change is possible NOW. Indeed, as Leo Tolstoy (1885/2016) reminded us, "Now […] is the only time when we have any power." Unless you're under 18, you're not going to have a different childhood, and the future isn't here yet. Not only is there no time like the present – there is actually no time but the present! (see Hoyt, 1990/2017; Rosenbaum, 2014)[1].

---

1 As St. Augustine (354–430 C.E.; quoted in Boscolo & Bertrando, 1993, p. 34) observed in his *Confessions*: "What is by now evident and clear is that neither future nor past exists, and it is inexact language to speak of three times – past, present, and future. Perhaps it would be exact to say: there are three times, a present of things past, a present of things present, a present of things to come. In the soul there are these three aspects of time, and I do not see them anywhere else. The present considering the past is the memory; the present considering the future is expectation." Indeed, there is really no time but NOW – as Dante Alighieri said in *The Divine Comedy* (c. 1265–1321), "Everywhere is here and every when is now." And Jorge Luis Borges (1947/1964, p. 234) wrote: "Time is the substance I am made of. Time is a river which sweeps me along, but I am the river; it is a tiger which destroys me, but I am the tiger; it is a fire which consumes me, but I am the fire." Octavio Paz (1963, pp. 124–125) said: "Yesterday is today, tomorrow is today, today everything is today." Nikos Kazantzakis (1965, p. 478) similarly noted: "No other moment exists: before and behind this moment is Nothing." American singer-songwriter Billy Joe Shaver (2009) exhorted us to "Live forever now." For more, see Hoyt (1990/2017, "On Time in Brief Therapy").

DOI: 10.4324/9781003468547-2

2. Approach each single session one-at-a-time (OAAT), each visit an episode or event complete unto itself (although more sessions might occur in the future, with the recognition that "one-at-a-time" doesn't necessarily mean "only one time").

3. The session is largely driven by the client's goals and skills (although the therapist may clarify goals and also contribute skills and resources as well as help identify those of the client). "Could it be," as Frank and Frank (1991, p. 149) asked, "that patients wished to spend less time in therapy than therapists?"

4. Constructive minimalism, that is, focusing therapeutically on what will help the client NOW rather than on diagnostic assessment (Talmon, 2018).

For many people, these basic ideas involve making fundamental shifts from conventional assumptions about therapy to a single session thinking and practice mindset:

1. From the idea that therapy must take a long time and that we should proceed slowly to the idea that change can occur NOW. Parkinson's Law – work expands or contracts to fill the time available for it – may influence how much and how fast clients benefit from psychotherapy (Appelbaum, 1975). SST/OAAT conveys the message that "the time to hesitate is through" and that NOW is the time to make changes. In his Foreword to Talmon's *Single Session Therapy*, Jerome Frank (1990) wrote about how the idea of making changes in one session challenges a lot of the assumptions/mindsets that many therapists have had: the beliefs that you have to gradually form an alliance, that you have to gradually uncover the underlying schemas or neuroses, that you then have to gradually work your way through or there will be too much resistance. When a regulatory board, as an expression of a long-term therapy mindset, tried to deny SST hours as credits toward psychologist licensure by contending that a single session could not be psychotherapy, Karen Young and Joseph Jebreen (2020) thoroughly debunked the wrongheaded effort. The belief that "one session can't really be therapy" is an ideological position cloaked in theory, not a reflection of the actual abundant research that supports SST. As Slive and Bobele (2019, p. 16) noted: "In an era of a well-intentioned focus on evidence-based practices, it is ironic that the evidence that supports SST is unknown to or ignored by many professionals." Rubin Battino (2014) cogently titled a paper, "Expectation: The Essence of Very Brief Therapy." There are both

placebo effects and *nocebo* effects – when the positive expectations or the negative expectations of the client (or clinician) regarding a treatment cause the treatment to have a more positive or negative effect than it otherwise would. As a wise person once said, whether a person thinks he or she is going to be a success or a failure – he or she is probably right!
    and

2. From the idea that it is the expert therapist who determines what is wrong and how to fix it, to the idea that the client is competent and capable and, perhaps with some facilitation, can solve problems. As Bill O'Hanlon and Michele Weiner-Davis (1989) put it in the title of their book, *In Search of Solutions: A New Direction in Psychotherapy*. I recall in a conversation with Steve de Shazer and John Weakland (Hoyt, 2001, p. 11) Steve's remark that "[Many therapists] are not 'mental health,' they're actually 'mental illness' professionals. It's not a mental health industry, it's a mental illness industry." We do have expertise, but so does the client – and it's his/her/their life! Clinicians can sometimes offer useful information, but I think Chris Iveson (2011, p. 121) said it well when he wrote: "Taking the radical position that we cannot know (or prescribe) the 'right' way forward for our clients, we have to trust their knowledge and treat them as the only experts in their own lives."

How and where you look influences what you see, and what you see influences what you do, 'round and around. Our mindset – our basic guiding beliefs – shapes the "lenses" (Hoffman, 1990/1993) through which we see the world and ourselves. Much traditional psychotherapy training inculcates beliefs that clients are not capable (that's why they're "patients") and that the therapist is "The Expert" on what is required and that we should proceed slowly and gradually. Economics that reward us for long-term therapy reinforce this mindset. And these mindset beliefs are not only held by therapists. We've all seen television programs in which the patient is endlessly "in treatment" and newspaper and magazine cartoon images of therapy that depict a patient laying on a couch. They teach the public long-term therapy prophecies. That's why the term <u>Single</u> Session Therapy is so powerful – as Jeff Young (2018) wrote, it is "in your face" and disruptive of the usual "go slow" mindset.

Regarding *client mindset*, Milton Erickson said: "Patients have problems because their conscious programming has too severely limited their capacities. The solution is to help them break through the limitations of their conscious attitudes to free their unconscious potential for problem solving" (Erickson, Rossi, & Rossi, 1976, p. 18); and "The patient comes to you with a certain mental set and they expect you to get into that set. If you surprise them, they let loose of their mental set and you can frame another mental set for them" (Erickson et al., 1976, p. 128; also see Hoyt & Battino, 2022). This is consistent with the concept of *destabilization*, as described by Dan Short (2021, pp. 286–287):

> Destabilization is defined as a momentary disruption of stable psychological patterns to encourage flexibility and learning. Therapeutic destabilization can be experienced in the form of doubt, uncertainty, surprise, shock, or confusion. [...] Therapeutic destabilization is needed only when it is necessary to circumvent a deeply established belief or rigid behavioral pattern.

Bill O'Hanlon's (2003) Inclusive Therapy approach (which highlights the use of permission, inclusion of opposites, and inclusion of exceptions) also disrupts and circumvents nonproductive mindsets.

Jeff Young (2018, pp. 46–50) identifies four common misunderstandings of SST:

- Misunderstanding #1: SST is seen as a specific model of therapy rather than a model of service delivery
- Misunderstanding #2: SST is described as a brief therapy rather than responding to clients' natural help-seeking behavior[2]
- Misunderstanding #3: SST is only suitable for clients facing simple problems
- Misunderstanding #4: SST means one session.

The renowned strategic therapist Jay Haley also thought that criticisms of SST were shortsighted and misguided. As Len Sperry (2010, p. 79) commented in a collection of Haley's papers: "It is particularly noteworthy that in later years, Haley favored 'rapid recoveries' and 'single-session therapies.'" Haley's appreciation for the potential of an SST can be seen in statements such as these:

> At one time short-term therapists were on the defensive. Long-term therapists thought of themselves as 'deep' and were confident, even arrogant. They liked to imply that brief therapy was a shallow, superficial endeavor. Brief therapists had to quote scientific outcome

---

2   Thus, by frequently choosing to come for one session, it was clients/patients – not therapists – who actually "invented" SST! Researchers have endeavored to identify which clients are most likely to find one session helpful and sufficient and what happens in a session to increase the likelihood of benefit, so that effective SST methods can be developed for more people.

results to prove their success, pointing out that research did not show any correlation between length of therapy and successful outcome.

—Jay Haley (1990, p. 4. 'Why Not Long-Term Therapy?')

We once assumed that long-term therapy was the base from which all therapy was to be judged. Now it appears that therapy of a single interview could become the standard for estimating how long and how successful therapy should be.

– Jay Haley (1993, back cover endorsement of M. Talmon, *Single Session Solutions: A Guide to Practical, Effective, and Affordable Therapy*)

and

Maybe you don't have a case really, except for the first interview. That would be nice, I think. Every therapist should shoot for one session.

—Jay Haley and Madeleine Richeport-Haley (2003, *The Art of Strategic Therapy*, p. 33)

Along similar lines, Jessica Schleider (2024, p. 85) writes in her book *Little Treatments, Big Effects*:

A single-session 'mindset' involves a set of guiding beliefs, present within the therapist or intervention and explicitly conveyed to the client. Any clinical encounter is understood as a singular event, because (1) something good can come from any one session, and (2) and one session could be the last. To establish this mindset within therapist-delivered SSIs [Single Session Interventions[3]], Hoyt and colleagues suggest beginning sessions with some variant of the following (and indeed, we follow these guidelines in providing our SSIs for people on psychotherapy waiting lists): 'Many people who come here and talk about their problems find that just one time can help a lot ... I'm willing to work hard today to help you get a better handle on things. Does that sound like something you'd like to do?' This framing establishes a shared expectation that change, even in this very brief period of time, is absolutely possible.

---

3   Schleider (2024, p. 52) explains: "My research group has since expanded this early definition, using a similar lens to Talmon's, but including delivery models made possible by technological advances (e.g., digital, self-administered programmes that do not involve a trained therapist). In this vein, we offer an updated definition of SSIs as 'specific, structured programmes that intentionally involve just one visit or encounter with a clinic, provider or programme.' [...] In short, SSIs create a new treatment access for youth experiencing mental illness, carrying particular benefit those who might otherwise go without support."

Aspects of Mindset

Discussing "The Single Session Mindset" and the possibility of clients returning for another session (or sessions), Monte Bobele and Arnie Slive (2014, pp. 97–98) offer this useful image:

> We do not conduct any session as if there will be another session. In other words, we do *one session at a time*. We prefer to think of walk-in therapy as a solitary pearl. Pearls begin as a solution to an oyster's problem. The formation of a pearl has a beginning, a middle, and a point where it is complete. If a jeweler anticipated making a long string of pearls, then each one is understood as related to, connected to, the one before and the one to come. Therapy is a lot like this process. [...] We encourage therapists to always consider the session as the creation of a solitary pearl. Of course another session may have occurred before the current one, and other sessions may follow, but the current session is complete and stands on its own.

Thus, Katy Stephenson (2023, p. 30) writes: "Single-session therapy is a process NOT one event." Hoyt (2014/2017, pp. 284–285) similarly comments:

> Effective single-session therapy helps people organize and catalyze, integrate and motivate, so that they can better access their own resources. [...] Our primary therapeutic effort and expertise should be directed toward encouraging, eliciting, evoking, exploring, and elaborating whatever the client brings that can be helpful to get them to where they want to go.

Federico Piccirilli and Lara Ermini (2021, pp. 59–60) note:

> The single-session mindset does not only work in vertical therapeutic processes: it can also be used in a horizontal therapy process. [*Horizontal*, like a string of pearls, refers to the traditional concept of psychotherapy which views a series of sessions as consecutive (first, second, third, fourth, etc.) whereas *vertical* refers to psychotherapy that develops in a single session complete in itself.] For example, with someone who decides to return after the first session, or who started therapy a while ago, therapists can approach each encounter as complete in itself. Its completeness, structure, strength, and coherence not only enable that single meeting to be useful, but also complete and cohesive, capable of standing alone.

SST involves seeking a pragmatic and parsimonious solution for the problem presented by the person. As Talmon (1993, p. 73) has described, this way of thinking, in which the search for psychohealth replaces the search for psychopathology, represents an alternative to the traditional model in psychiatry and psychotherapy. Focusing on *what works* is usually better, in therapy as in life. Psychiatrist Anne Lutz (2014) and many others have written about the profound shift and "new direction" (O'Hanlon & Weiner-Davis, 1989) entailed in interviewing to identify strengths and resources rather than focusing on symptoms and weaknesses.

Concerning "The Vital Role of the Therapist's Mindset," Flavio Cannistrà (2021, p. 77) wrote:

> How we look – which is directed by our mindset – influences what we see, and what we see influences how we proceed. This [...] is about mindset, but also about epistemological and trans-theoretical matters. My meta-intention is that the reader becomes more aware of how our mindset shapes clinical reasoning processes, the logic within how we listen and how we speak, the choice and clarification of the words we use, and thus, how we work with our clients – and how we may help them in a single session.

He notes that different theories predict (foretell in advance) different lengths of treatment, that different theories operate from different observations and opinions, and that (2021, p. 85) "a choice must be made. Actually, a choice is always made. Here, I present my choices to be briefer in therapy" and then enumerates choices to be pragmatic, to be efficient, to avoid theory reification, and to adopt a multi-theoretical mindset.

In a subsequent paper, "The Single Session Therapy Mindset: Fourteen Principles Gained Through an Analysis of the Literature," Cannistrà (2022, p. 2) notes that it is essential to take mindset into account because "the organized series of ways in which we think and practice acts as a guide to a number of key points of the therapy itself." He quotes others who have also referenced the cardinal significance of mindset, such as:

- "Man operates with a set of premises about the phenomena he perceives and [...] his interaction with reality in the widest sense [...] will be determined by these premises" (Watzlawick, Beavin, & Jackson, 1967, p. 262).
- "A crucial element for conducting walk-in [single] sessions is the therapist's own beliefs about the effectiveness of brief therapy.

Therapists' expectations are communicated overtly and covertly about how rapid and how much change can be expected" (Slive & Bobele, 2012, p. 29).

- "SST can be thought of more as an affirmative and optimistic mindset [...] rather than as a particular method" (Hoyt, 2021, p. 31).
- "The 'DNA' of good SST [includes] mobilizing so-called 'client and extra-therapeutic factors' such as the client's underlying strengths, supportive elements in the environment, and chance events of spontaneous healing. [...] The single session therapist believes that the client has resources and that these are part of the therapy" (Talmon, 2014, p. 35).

Cannistrà then goes on to review numerous contributions and insightfully explicates fourteen principles of a single session mindset:

1. A single session may be enough.
2. The therapist can play an active role.
3. People have resources they can use to feel better.
4. The client is the expert in their own life.
5. Different methods may be used.
6. Further sessions may be needed.
7. SST is suitable for different contexts and needs.
8. It's fine to aim for small or simple interventions.
9. It's fine to have less prior knowledge.
10. It's best to stick with process and the here and now.
11. Results are mainly achieved outside the session.
12. A structure is needed for the single session.
13. A client-therapist relationship can be established rapidly.
14. Nothing is taken for granted.

Sam Porter and Tim Pitt (2023) defined the single session mindset this way:

A core set of beliefs and attitudes (about people, therapy, and change), which are intentionally embraced and enacted, before and during single session work, in order to align the therapist and the client toward the possibility of creating change within a single session.

Based on interviews they conducted with many leading experts in the SST field, Porter and Pitt identified nine core beliefs (which overlap those listed above):

1.   Clients are the experts in their own life.
2.   Clients have strengths and resources to make things better.
3.   People are always changing.
4.   One session can be enough.
5.   The therapist should play an active role in creating a sense of hope within the client to maximize each therapeutic encounter.
6.   Every session should have a beginning, middle, and end.
7.   Treat the person and their situation, not their diagnosis.
8.   The therapist just needs to get the client moving.
9.   Change occurs in different forms.

One Size Doesn't Fit All

Erickson said (quoted in Haley, 1973, p. 291): "I would want to improve it in a very minor way. As soon as I got the slightest minor change in it, the way would be open for a larger change." Haley (1982, p. 23) agreed: "The small change invariably led to the larger one. As Erickson put it, if you want a large change you should ask for a small one." Ericksonians (see Short, Erickson, & Klein, 2005) call this *progression*: do it just a little bit different, then a little bit more different, building incrementally on a small change. Get a foot in the door. A small change can lead to a big change. I once heard John Weakland, who was part of the MRI group, say in an interview to somebody who had brought up something that was going to be a distraction, "Would it be okay with you if we solve the problem and then if we still have time, and you're interested in that, we can come back to that?" (See Gergen & Gergen, 1984, on the distinction between *progressive, regressive, stabilizing,* and *digressive* narratives.) It was brilliant. He didn't say, "Don't waste my time" or "You're going sideways" or "Aren't you just trying to deflect and avoid?" Just "Would it be okay if we solve the problem, and then if there's time left, we'd come back to that?" It was very elegant – we're trying to get from here to there, not these other places. His guiding mindset was to stay focused on the desired goal.

Our mindset and psychotherapy theories direct us toward different time orientations, toward focusing on the past, the present, or the future. All may be useful, but as Erickson (1954b, p. 127) reminded us, "Emphasis should be placed more upon what the patient does in the present and will do in the future than upon a mere understanding of why some long-past event occurred." Thus, as Giorgio Nardone and Paul Watzlawick (1990, 2005) and others have noted, we need to address how *in the present* the client is staying "stuck."

In our 2023 book, *Brief Therapy Conversations: Exploring Efficient Intervention in Psychotherapy*, Flavio Cannistrà and I (Hoyt & Cannistrà, 2023, p. 66) also had this colloquy:

FLAVIO: So, we said a lot; is there anything else you want to say about mindset?

MICHAEL: Be flexible. You don't want your mindset to be so set that it can't change. It's mindset, not mind-set-in-concrete.

FLAVIO: Maybe more than mindset, we have to talk about mind-*setting*.

MICHAEL: Yeah, that's a good way to look at it, as a verb, 'mind-setting.' The basic mindset in brief therapy is: *Change is possible now or soon.* 'You have an ability that I can help you recognize. Once you know what your goal is, you will be able to use your abilities. We can talk about how you're going to achieve your goal.'

It's good to *pay attention to what you pay attention to*. How we make sense of our worlds – the stories we tell ourselves and each other – does much to determine what we experience, our actions and our destinies. Some stories are better than others because they are more enlivening and encouraging, helping people to get more of what they want. They carry wisdom and hope. They open people's hearts and touch their feelings. They speak to the person's truth or dream. They tap into our strengths and resources. They invigorate us, making us feel more alive and more deeply human. How we look influences what we see, and what we see influences what we do, 'round and around. What you focus on tends to grow, so be mindful of your mindset, your language, and what you choose to emphasize.

You might ask a client: "When you're walking out, when your hand is on the door and you're about to leave, what do you want to be taking with you?" If you frame it the right way, most people will go, "Yeah, I'd like to have some ideas of what the next steps are that I should take regarding the problem that brought me here." I think there are certain people, however, who come in wanting to have a longer-term relationship, they want ongoing support as they sort out how they got to be who they are and engage in extended self-exploration. They've been inculcated: their mindset is "I have to explore my whole childhood and we'll talk all about that stuff." And there are other people who come in much more focused – they have a particular problem and they want a specific solution.

As Haley (1990, p. 10) wrote:

> Long-term therapy is usually defended with the argument that the client is fragile and needs support in meeting life's problems. In contrast,

the brief therapist tends to have the view that all the person needs to become normal like other people is a few sessions to straighten out some problems. The underlying premise of brief therapy is fundamentally different from the long-term view of the human condition and how people cope with it.

Some people don't want to come in because they think it's going to be sort of the fly-paper model: Once you land, you can't get out again. And you're going to have to go through every bloody miserable thing in your life and all of that. When I was preparing to do an SST workshop with the clinical staff at a large police department in California, I was talking with the chief police psychologist and I said:

> I know a lot of the problems that the police have, when they come to see a therapist, they have pretty heavy problems, they've had traumas and seen horrible things, and I'm not sure whether or how often everything's going to get dealt with in one session. [See, for example, Mitchell & Dorian, 2017; and Kirschman, Kamena, & Fay, 2014.] And he said, 'No, of course not, but you know, as the risk of stereotyping, most of the police who will come to see a therapist, most are relatively young, male, action-oriented, pragmatic, they're problem solvers. They don't want to spend a lot of time talking about how they have a feeling about how their mother was and how their father was, they want to get some ideas of what to do, so I think they would be ideal candidates for a very brief therapy, if someone could equip them with some of those skills. And if they need to do more, they will do more.'

Another time, I was before a large audience and a woman stood up and asked, "What group is best for brief therapy? Men or women and which race or ethnic group?" I thought and then said,

> I wouldn't look at it that way. I'd think of it much more as what do they want? And is there something within their grasp, maybe with a little help, they can get pointed towards some of their own skills, and maybe get some extra ideas from the therapist. It's not, is this or that better for Caucasians or Asians or Blacks or Latinos, men or women, etc. That's not the way to think of it. It's much more useful to be looking for what resources the person has. And it's going to be different in different cultures. So if someone is coming from a collectivist culture, talking about how their

family could help them is going to be very different; whereas, if someone is coming from a more individualized culture, talking a lot about 'Well, how will your uncle feel?' maybe isn't going to be as useful as 'How can you be more strong and independent, stand on your own?'

One size doesn't fit all. Rather than having just one approach for everyone, or for everyone from a certain group, it is important to tailor interventions to fit the person. A good meta-mindset is "Our primary therapeutic effort and expertise should be directed toward encouraging, eliciting, evoking, exploring, and elaborating whatever the client brings that can be helpful to get them where they want to go" (Hoyt, 2014, p. 69). Cultural aspects will be discussed further in Chapter 6, but I don't think it's useful to have the mindset that single session or very brief therapy is better for one group or another.

Therapist Resistances to Brief (and Single Session) Therapy

Many years ago, when I first began to study and then teach methods of brief and short-term therapy, I encountered – first in myself, then in others – a series of concerns and objections that I came to call "therapist resistances to short-term therapy" (Hoyt, 1985/1995). Each "resistance" is actually a response to violating the "go slow" and related mindsets of conventional long-term psychotherapy. Remembering the psychodynamic principle that it can be helpful to get a more open mind by identifying potential resistances, here is an annotated list:

1. *The belief that "more is better."* Actually, *better* is better. Too much is too much – think of vitamin (or alcohol) overdoses. Shakespeare counseled (in *King John*, Act 4, Scene 2): "To paint the lily [...] is wasteful and ridiculous excess."[4] In 167 C.E., in his *Meditations*, Marcus Aurelius also wrote:

---

4   The actual reference from the play, *King John* (Act 4, Scene 2):

> To gild refined gold, to paint the lily
> To throw a perfume on the violet
> To smooth the ice, or add another hue
> Unto the rainbow, or with taper-light
> To seek the beauteous eye of heaven to garnish,
> Is wasteful and ridiculous excess.

In *King Lear* (Act I, Scene 4), Shakespeare also said: "Striving to better, oft we mar what's well."

> Ever run the short way; and the short way is the way of nature, with perfect soundness in each word and deed as the goal. Such an aim will give you freedom from anxiety and strife, and from all compromise and artifice.

2. *The myth of the "pure gold" of analysis.* It is good to remember that in his last great paper, "Analysis Terminable and Interminable," Freud (1937/1964) advised that analysis goes on and on and you can always analyze – but it doesn't always help people. He recommended "alloying the pure gold of analysis" with other metals to make a more durable and efficient therapeutic instrument – suggestion, guidance, education, encouragement. He talked with people and sometimes gave them reassurance and advice. Still, in some circles, "long-term" and "deep" are seen as the gold standard, whilst other approaches are dismissed as "superficial" or "palliative."

3. *Belief in the inappropriateness of greater therapist activity.* This gets at Jerome Frank's (1990) comments about the traditional assumptions of long-term therapy, that we need to always go gradually to build alliance and avoid stimulating resistance.

4. *The confusion of patients' and therapists' interests.* Most folks who seek therapy have a particular problem they want help with; but we therapists tend to want to explore and look for other issues. Indeed, there is even the concept of "flight into health," the idea that someone should be restrained from improving too quickly. I remember Steve de Shazer and John Weakland (in Hoyt, 2001b, pp. 7–8 and p. 14) laughing about that one.

5. *Financial (and other) pressures.* There is the need to keep our billable hours booked, and there are also other rewards for holding on to particular clients: we like them, we enjoy the pleasures of intimate conversations, we want to see how things work out.

6. *Countertransference and termination problems.* The need to be needed, the tendency to project our issues on to clients to see how they handle them, and difficulties saying goodbye. As Neil Sedaka's 1960 hit song said, "Breaking Up Is [Sometimes] Hard to Do."

7. *Psychological reactance.* There is the interesting phenomenon (Brehm, 1966) that we tend to value something more if we're told that we can't have it. Therapists may object if told that they have to assist someone quickly, *even if it helps!*

8. *Paperwork.* Finishing cases quickly and efficiently leads to starting new cases, with required additional intake forms, paperwork, possible authorization requests, etc. It may not be in the best interests of the

clients we're supposed to serve, but it is often easier (for the therapist) to simply write: "Continue therapy – return in one week." SST can also be burdensome if therapists who offer SST appointments also have to continue seeing the same number of regular intake appointments (Robinson, Harvey, McDonald, & Honegger, 2021, p. 145)

Context of Competence

To my mind, there is a "Context of Competence" that we co-create with clients, in which effective therapy – in one session, or more – takes place.[5] The Venn diagram shown in Figure 2.1 depicts three overlapping circles, labeled ALLIANCE/GOALS/RESOURCES. Therapy takes place where the three intersect. If you have GOALS and an ALLIANCE but don't access RESOURCES, nothing happens. If you have RESOURCES and an ALLIANCE, but don't have GOALS, there's nothing to do, no direction; if the client could match up their GOALS and RESOURCES on their own, they wouldn't need the therapist. Hence, all three are needed: the *Context of Competence* is where GOALS and RESOURCES come together through the ALLIANCE. The work is collaborative. Effective therapy, one session or otherwise, involves all three (Hoyt, 2017, p. 300).

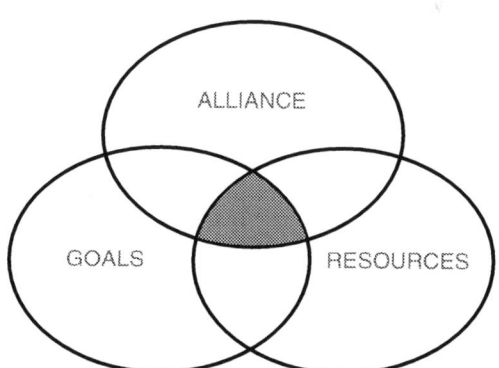

Figure 2.1 Context of Competence

Source: From M.F. Hoyt, 2014. ©M.F. Hoyt. Used with permission.

---

5   Yasmin Ajmal (2001, p. 13), introducing solution-focused thinking, has also referred to "creating a context of competence." She wrote (pp. 14–15): "Listening out for strengths and helping someone to build a helpful description of themselves can be a powerful starting point for change. [...] The skill is to listen out for anything that might be helpful and to persist, gently, in the belief that the person does bring something positive to their situation."

I use the term *resources* here in a broad, generic sense, to refer to whatever skills, capacities, abilities, and competencies the client (and therapist) may have that they can apply toward resolving the problem(s) that have led the client to seek therapeutic help. Others may be more specific. Dryden (2019, p. 73), for example, has written: "In my view 'strengths' are factors that are internal to the person and can be distinguished from 'resources' that are external to the person." This granular differentiation may help guide client and clinician where to look. Discussing the importance of resource talk, Elliott Connie and Adam Froerer (2023, p. 166) write:

> People don't often think about their resources, and as they learn to identify them, they'll realize their own capacity for greatness, which they need in order to achieve change. [...] The fact that the clients who walk into your office have lived as long as they have, no matter their age, is evidence that they have resources.

I also prefer the term GOALS rather than PROBLEMS. Clients will tell you about their problems and difficulties, but you don't want to stop there – as George et al. (1990) nicely put it, the focus needs to move from "problem to solution." It's "solution talk" (Furman & Ahola, 1992) and "resource talk" (Connie & Froerer, 2023) that makes a difference that leads to change. Techniques follow from your mindset. They give therapist and client a focus, helping them to see and use whatever the client's (and therapist's) relevant resources may be.

It is important to keep in mind that the therapeutic alliance involves *being allies for a purpose*. Bordin (1979; also see Norcross, 2011) identified three components to the therapeutic alliance (sometimes called the *therapeutic relationship* or the *working alliance*): tasks, goals, and bond. If you identify Goals (or Problems) and have an Alliance but don't access Resources, nothing happens. If you have an Alliance and access Resources but don't consider Goals / Problems, you may have a pleasant relationship, but there's nothing to do – maybe a friendly visit, but what's the purpose? If the client could match up his / her / their Goals and Resources on their own, bringing to bear skills and competencies to deal with problems, they probably wouldn't be in your office. The *Context of Competence* is where the client is helped to bring resources and goals together via the therapeutic alliance. All three are often required.

It will be useful to consider, in the chapters that follow, how a Context of Competence is created and used in SST.

The Practice of SST

3

The first session is of prime importance. It is both the beginning and sets the direction for further work. As Aristotle said, "A good start is half the job." In English we also have the saying, "As the twig is bent, so grows the tree." In *The First Session in Brief Therapy*, my colleagues Simon Budman, Steven Friedman, and I (1992) asked practitioners of different theoretical orientations to each write a chapter illustrating their work in a typical first session. Looking across the different approaches, we found that first sessions – including but not limited to those when the first session was offered as an SST – that led to successful therapies generally have these common characteristics:

1. Establish rapport
2. Define purpose of meeting, orienting client on how to use therapy
3. Create opportunities for client to express thoughts, feelings, behaviors
4. Assess the client's problems, strengths, motivation, expectations, and goals
5. Evaluate possible psychiatric complaints when indicated, including suicide risk and alcohol/drug abuse when appropriate
6. Mutually (therapist and client) formulate a treatment plan
7. Make initial treatment interventions and assess their effects
8. Suggest/assign "homework" or other tasks as appropriate
9. Define treatment parameters, either a number ("up to 10 sessions") or "only as long as necessary"
10. Make future appointments as needed
11. Handle fees and payments.

DOI: 10.4324/9781003468547-3

Around the same time, Moshe Talmon, Bob Rosenbaum, and I were investigating what might be accomplished when the client was offered the possibility that "the first session might be the last." As noted in Chapter 1, after reviewing the literature and doing a retrospective examination of 200 one-session cases seen in our clinic, we did a prospective study of 58 cases and found that the majority (58.6%) elected to finish therapy in one session even though more sessions were available.

Building on our Chapter 2 examination of an SST/OAAT mindset, here we highlight some relative indications and contraindications for the likelihood of successful SST. This will set the stage for further discussion of guideline steps and SST/OAAT practices. What follows has been adapted and expanded from Talmon (1990, 1993), Rosenbaum, Hoyt, and Talmon (1990), Hoyt, Rosenbaum, and Talmon (1992), and Hoyt (1990/2017, 1994a/1995, 2000a, 2017). In addition to his many original contributions, some of the same points have been echoed and elaborated by Dryden (e.g., 2017, 2018, 2019b, 2021, 2022), an expert rational emotive behavior therapy (REBT) practitioner (see Chapter 4, p. 79) who has described his enthusiasm (2019b, p. xi) when reading and re-reading Talmon (1990) – and then Hoyt and Talmon (2014) and Hoyt et al. (2018) – and discovering the world of SST.

What Are the Relative Indications and Contraindications for Successful SST?

Although sometimes people with seemingly "easy" or "simple" problems may not find SST adequate, whereas others with seemingly more "difficult" or "complex" problems will find benefit in one (or a few) sessions, based on our research and subsequent clinical experience (as well as that of others), those who in general are more likely to benefit from SST include:

- Clients who come to solve a specific problem for which a solution is in their control.[1]

---

1   Writing from an object-relations psychodynamic perspective, Michael Stadter (1996, p. 226) reports a clinical example of a single-session therapy he did with a woman ("Katrina") who was angry about a situation in her workplace. Although noting several areas in which he would have liked to have done more therapy had there been more time, he acknowledges (p. 232): "However, from her standpoint the single-session therapy was very successful; she obtained what she wanted. I need to respect that (and keep my own narcissism in check)." He goes on (p. 232): "Katrina evidenced all three of Hoyt and colleagues' (1992) key factors in single session therapy. First, we quickly established a good working alliance. Second, while she began the session feeling she could do nothing to improve the situation, she quickly became engaged in the process of looking at what she *could* do. [...] Lastly, she was *ready!*"

- Clients who essentially need reassurance that their reaction to a troubling situation is normal. "I'd be surprised and worried if you *didn't* feel that way, given what you've been through" can be a normalizing and very useful statement.

- Clients seen with significant others or family members who can serve as natural supports and "co-therapists" (and, if needed, a social context that may be reinforcing and perpetuating a problem can be addressed).[2]

- Clients who can identify (perhaps with the therapist's assistance) helpful solutions, past successes, and exceptions to the problem.

- Clients who have a particularly "stuck" feeling (e.g., anger, guilt, grief) toward a past event.

- Clients who come for evaluation and need referral to medical or other services (e.g., legal, vocational, financial, religious counseling).

- Clients who are likely to be better off without any treatment, such as "spontaneous improvers," "non-responders," and those for whom an extended therapeutic relationship is likely to have a "negative therapeutic reaction" (Frances & Clarkin, 1981).

- Clients faced with a truly insoluble situation that can be recast in terms of goals that can be productively addressed. For example, a man who had gone from physician to physician and therapist to therapist looking for someone who could fix his badly Alzheimer-afflicted parent ("How about hypnosis? Would magnets or megavitamins help?") finally found help when the focus was shifted to the therapy of acceptance, grieving and coping, and reality-based problem solving.

And, in contradistinction, those for whom SST is less likely to be adequate include:

- Clients who might require inpatient care (e.g., acutely suicidal or psychotic).

---

2   The idea of a systemic-interactional perspective is not new. Hippocrates (c. 460–377 B.C.E.), in *Aphorisms of His School* (quoted in Calvin, 1986, p. 472) counseled: "Life is short, the Art Long, opportunity fleeting, experience treacherous, judgment difficult. The physician must be ready, not only to do his duty himself, but also to secure the cooperation of the patient, of the attendants, and of externals."

Seneca the Younger (c. 4 B.C.E.-C.E. 65), in *On the Shortness of Life* (quoted in Costa, 2005, pp. 1–2), also gave advice that emphasized the SST message to "seize the moment," maximize the effect of the first (and often only) session, and get on with it: "Hence the dictum of the greatest of doctors: 'Life is short, art is long.' [...] It is not that we have a short time to live, but that we waste a lot of it. Life is long enough, and a sufficiently generous amount has been given to us for the highest achievements if it were all well invested [...] Why do we complain about nature? She has acted kindly: life is long if you know how to use it."

- Clients seeking relief from symptoms that suggest a strong biological or chemical component (e.g., schizophrenia, manic-depression, active alcohol and/or other drug addiction) as well as those evincing so-called severe personality disorders. Major mental illness and personality disorders are very unlikely to get resolved completely in one visit, but keep in mind that such folks also have a condition called "life" and may benefit from SST to help solve specific problems. Normalizing and successfully assisting clients to deal with quotidian concerns may also perhaps encourage them to take an important step toward further resolution of underlying conditions.
- Clients who request long-term therapy up front, including those who are anticipating and have prepared for prolonged self-exploration. (At a workshop I might make a face and facetiously say "Hi, I'm Michael. Here's my genogram. I'd like to come every Tuesday at 10 a.m. for the next year.") Folks wanting long-term therapy may need to shift their mindset to specific problem solving in order to find SST satisfaction.
- Clients who need ongoing support to work through (and escape) the effects of childhood and/or adult abuse. Don't blame them! Many abuse sufferers may have relationship reluctance, and some will like the in-and-out OAAT of SST whereas others will need more time to meaningfully engage and may not find SST adequate.
- Clients with longstanding eating disorders or severe OCD, as well as those with chronic pain syndromes and somatoform disorders.

Quick (1996, pp. 176–177) concurs:

> [A] number of different types of clients [are] likely to benefit from a single session. One type includes people who present with a specific problem for which a situation is within their control. A little problem solving, brainstorming, and clarification can make a big difference. Other clients who make excellent use of a single appointment are those who are experiencing normal reactions to loss, stress, or life transition. Reassurance about the normalcy and appropriateness of one's response can bring great relief. For other people, a single session provides the opportunity for referral to specific resources other than psychotherapy. Clients who have not yet utilized nonpsychotherapy support and community resources generally can be encouraged to do so before engaging in more psychotherapy. [Moreover] sometimes more extensive treatment can exacerbate the very problem the client is seeking to eliminate, and preventing additional treatment can be of value. This can occur when a normal transition is labeled as

pathological. [...] Treatment can also make things worse if it creates or maintains an illusion that an unresolvable problem can be resolved. [...] As Chubb and Evans (1985) point out, continuing open-ended therapy can engender a false hope or sense of security that simply 'being in therapy' will take care of the problem. Clarifying that risk may be the most effective intervention the therapist can provide.

Keep in mind that these are general attitudes and relative indications/contraindications.

An SST may start or extend, but not necessarily complete, resolution of severe problems. As quoted in one of the epigraphs that open this book, Lao Tzu (Chinese philosopher, 6th century B.C.E.) said, "The journey of a thousand miles begins with a single step." Emphasize abilities and strengths rather than pathology, asking "How can this client create a solution?" rather than stopping at "How does this patient create this problem?" (Rosenbaum et al., 1990/1995, p. 123). It is good to recall that the word *diagnosis* comes from the Greek and Latin words "dia" and "gnossis." "Dia" means "passing through" or "way" (like "via") and "gnossis" means "knowledge." So a useful "diagnosis" should point a way or give functional information that would actually help us help the client (Hoyt, 1995; Hoyt & Cannistrà, 2023a, pp. 28–29).

In Search of Solutions: Creative Application of the Following Clinical Guidelines Facilitates SST

1. *"Seed" change through induction and preparation.* Therapy and any needed assessment can be intertwined (Denner & Reeves, 1997). To help the client "hit the decks running" it can be useful to engage the person via a pre-session phone call or letter encouraging a focus on goals and collection of information about competencies, past successes, and exceptions to the problem. An efficacious technique can be de Shazer's (1985) generic skeleton key Formula First Session Task: "Between now and when we meet, I would like you to observe, so you can describe to me, what happens that you want to continue to happen." It could be helpful to know when the presenting problem is not present, or at least not so bad. For example, "It sounds like sometimes you have a full-blown panic attack, but other times you get nervous but don't completely freak-out – what's the difference?" *or* "From what you've said, sometimes you drink way too much, but other times you manage to stop before it's

too much – how do you do that when you manage to stop?" or "Some of the quarrels you and your partner have get really ugly, but other times you can disagree without it getting out of hand – what helps you to keep from going over the top?" (Such questions can also be asked, of course, in session and not just pre-session.)

Windy Dryden (2017, p. 127) describes a thoughtful pre-session telephone protocol, including items asking:

- *What made you decide that now is the right time for therapy?*
- *How do you think I can best help you to deal with the issue?*
- *What have you done that had helped with the issue?*
- *What strengths do you have as a person that you can use that might help you address the issue?*
- *I would like to know what your preferred way of learning is so that I can tailor the session to best help you. Can you help shed light on this?*
- *Is there anything you would like me to know that will help me prepare for our face-to-face session or that would help us get the most out of the session?*

At the Italian Center for Single Session Therapy (Cannistrà & Piccirilli, 2021c, p. 201; see De Grande, 2013, for some recent quantitative evidence for efficaciousness of pre-session preparation), a "SST Pre-Treatment Questionnaire" asks:

- *What is the goal you would like to achieve with today's session?*
- *How motivated do you feel to work on this goal?*
- *What characteristics and resources do you have which you think can help us achieve this goal?*
- *Think about whether in the last days / weeks you have noticed improvements, changes, or simply different behaviors which are in some ways helpful for overcoming the problem [...]*

In Holland, working in a corporate context, Helen Van Empel (2013, in press) offers online SST and advises SST clients how "to make the most of your session," including recommending:

- *Prior to the Session.* It is important to take the time to properly prepare in order to ensure maximum effectiveness. Consider the current situation and set clear goals for what you wish to achieve. Reflect on past efforts and the impact they had and consider any necessary adjustments to be made moving forward. By taking the time to properly prepare, you will be better equipped to achieve your desired results during the session.

Other pre-SST (phone call or online) questions to consider (some have been mentioned above):

- What's the problem (*or* concern *or* trouble)? What is the situation now? (psychiatric / medical / legal)?

- Who is the customer – who's most concerned? (see Coyne, 1987)
- What hidden agenda may there be? (Cummings & Sayama, 1995, remind us that in addition to an explicit agenda there may be an implicit agenda, such as wanting time off work or building a child custody case against an estranged spouse.)
- How and how soon does the client anticipate the problem will be solved?
- How does the client think therapy will be helpful in dealing with the problem?
- What made the client decide that now was the right time for therapy?
- Am I (therapist) the right person for this case? (Do I need to consult with someone about this particular problem? Working with this ethnic group?)

2. *Develop an alliance and co-create obtainable treatment goals.* As Talmon (2018, p. 149) commented: "The essence of any psychotherapy is the same as that of SST. It is based on the abilities of the therapist and patient to create a therapeutic alliance in the here-and-now of each therapeutic encounter."

When getting started, inquire about change since pretreatment contact and amplify accordingly (see Weiner-Davis, de Shazer, & Gingerich 1987). Introduce the possibility of one session being adequate and recruit the patient's cooperation. A typical opening might be something like:

> The purpose of today's meeting is to find out what brings you here and then to work on figuring out the next steps toward a solution. Experience shows that we may be able to do that in one meeting. If so, would you be interested in that?

As I wrote previously (Hoyt, 2018, p. 157):

> In our study at Kaiser, we implied and invited – 'Maybe in one visit; are you interested in that?' – but did not insist on a one-session format. Insistence produces resistance, imposition produces opposition, push produces pushback – so I think it is important to offer and invite, but not demand, one visit. In our studies of SST, we have been careful to refer to the 'POSSIBILITY of one session being enough' and to say 'When the first session MAY be the last.'

We want to be goal-directed as soon as feasible, but as Cannistrà notes (in Cannistrà & Piccirilli, 2021, p. 98), some clients may insist (at least at first) on being more problem-focused, complaining about what has bothered them. In such instances, it will not help to be what Nylund and Corsiglia (1994) called "solution-<u>forced</u>" (not focused). As Cannistrà advises:

> We believe that the best way to avoid making mistakes is to go with what clients consider most important: if they want a space to talk about the problem we should (while containing it) give them this opportunity. Aside from the issue of priorities, *defining a goal* remains essential. In the context of SST, a distinction must be drawn between the aim of the treatment and the aim of the session: while the former concerns what individuals generally expect from therapy, the latter is 'what should be achieved by the end of the appointment.' In our practice, we ask questions like: 'What is the goal you would like to have achieved by the time this session finishes?'

3. *Allow enough time.* Most of us work in the 50-minute hour, which is usually adequate but consider scheduling a longer session to allow for a complete process or intervention.

   Particularly with a couple or family, a 60–90-minute SST session may be helpful – you don't want to create an alliance and hear about the history and current situation and the clients' hopes and then, rather than talking about possible solutions, look at the clock and need to say, "We're out of time today – let's pick this up at our next meeting." Pam Rycroft and Jeff Young (2021, pp. 48–49) wisely counsel "make time your friend," using the temporal parameters to structure the session and organize priorities (e.g., "Given that we only have 20 minutes left, what do you think we should focus on so that you'll find today's meeting worthwhile?"). Make each moment count; don't waste time. As the other epigraph that opens this book says, "So teach us to number our days that we may get us a heart of wisdom" (Moses, *Psalms* 90: 12).

   "Brief therapy" and "Single Session Therapy" are defined not by a specific number of minutes, respectively, but rather by the attitude of making the most of whatever amount of time is allotted and available. The famed strategic hypnotherapist Milton Erickson preferred to have two-hour single sessions, explaining: "That is how long it takes to get something done!" (quoted in Rossi & Rossi, 2014, p. 233). For some discussions of therapy involving briefer sessions than the conventional 50–60 minutes, see Barten (1965), Castelnuovo-Tedesco (1986), Dreiblatt and Weatherly (1965), Koegler and Cannon (1966), Leibenluft, Tasman, and Green (1993), McNeilly (1994), Stone (2002), and Zirkle (1961). Chrystal Fullen (in Bobele et al., 2018, pp. 236–242) reports how when a client-couple arrived late, she and her co-therapist (Brittany Houston) realized that they still had "a whole 30 minutes" – and used the time very well. Thinking about time and therapy, here's a head-scratcher: Would Berenbaum's (1969) single ten-hour marathon session be considered a form of prolonged brief therapy or a brief prolonged therapy?

4. *Focus on "pivot chords," ambiguities that may facilitate transitions into different directions* (Rosenbaum et al., 1990/1995). Look for ways of meeting the client in his or her worldview while, at the same time, offering a new perspective – "reframing" introduces the possibility of seeing and/or acting differently. "Re-framing" essentially means "same facts, different meaning" (see Watzlawick et al., 1974; Bandler & Grinder, 1982; also see Coyne, 1985). As Steenbarger (2002, p. 671) wrote: "Even relatively small shifts in the map can produce new patterns of thinking, feeling, and acting that can assume a life of their own. This can be observed in the 'pivot chords' described by Robert Rosenbaum, Michael Hoyt, and Moshe Talmon, who use ambiguity in client verbalizations to open the door to new ways of construing problematic situations."

In one classic example (although he didn't use the term "reframing"), Harry Stack Sullivan (1954) told a bored and unhappy housewife that he found her complaints very encouraging because they indicated that she had intelligence and energy that needed to be better used. In another case, I met with a man who had made a feeble and unsuccessful suicide attempt in an effort to get an insurance settlement for his family. When I commented, "You know, in some ways you're a hero" he responded, "What do you mean 'a hero.' I'm such a f- up I couldn't even do that right." I asked, "Do you know the term 'dead-beat dad'?" He did: someone who runs away rather than being responsible and taking care of their kids and family. I then said, "That's why I said 'hero.' You're someone who would even give up your life to help your family. I'm not so sure about your technique, but your heart is in the right place." He got tearful (I did too) because we had identified and honored his good intention.[3] This led into a

---

3   A number of authors (e.g., Armstrong, 2015; Taibbi, 2016; Chow, 2018; Leslie, 2019), while not necessarily advocating for SST, all emphasize the importance of the first session being emotionally engaging so that the client comes away not just having been "assessed" at an "intake" but feeling encouraged and with new ideas and skills. Freud (1900) may have thought that dreams are the "royal road" (*via regia*) to the unconscious, but emotion is the rapid road to connection and change. No surprise that Joseph Campbell (1949), Carlos Castenada (1968), and Jack Kornfield (1993) all counseled to follow "a path with heart." (Note: the Latin root of the word *courage* is *cor*, which means "heart.") In her book, *Caste: The Origins of Our Discontents*, Pulitzer-Prize winner Isabel Wilkerson (2020, pp. 370–373) beautifully tells a story near the end (in a chapter titled "The Heart is the Last Frontier") in which she had to call a plumber to her home because of a bad water leak in the basement. Wilkerson is Black and the rude and seemingly racist white man

discussion of other ways he could help his family until he found a job. The "re-frame" went from "suicidal f- up" to "devoted self-sacrificing hero." He felt the one session had given him what he needed – encouragement and a new direction. He said he wasn't going to harm himself and that he didn't need another appointment but promised to call if he felt stuck. In another instance, meeting with a couple, when I pointed out that what one partner described as "overbearing" and "controlling" behavior was the other person's well-intended but perhaps heavy-handed attempts to be useful, the other person said "Yeah, I'm not trying to be a jerk; I just want to help" – and became much more open to hearing about other ways of acting that would be more helpful.

5. *Go slow and look for patient's strengths.* Too often we jump on the first thing we see (e.g., "You say you're depressed. You know, depression is often really anger turned inward. So, what are you angry about?") rather than taking the time (remember: we have a WHOLE session!) to see what else may be going on, what solutions have already been attempted, what may be the client's agenda and priorities, etc.

6. *Practice solutions experientially.* Rehearsing desired outcomes in the session provides a "glimpse of the future," teaches and reinforces useful skills, and inspires enthusiasm and movement. It may also allow, if the client gets "stuck," time to discuss and resolve difficulties that otherwise would impede progress. Milton Erickson advised (in Zeig, 1980, p. 72): "I believe that patients and students should do things. They learn better, remember better." Haley (1963, 1969, 1977, 1984) sought to bring about change not primarily by talking but via change in behavior. Social psychology research (see Collins & Hoyt, 1972; Hoyt, Henley, & Collins, 1972) also demonstrates that changes in behavior can result in changes in attitudes. Whatever the theoretical explanation – learning the words and behaviors, neuropsychology modification, "passing the test" and emotional relief by disconfirming unwarranted negative expectations (Budman & Hoyt, 1993), a "corrective emotional experience" (Alexander & French, 1946; Nardone & Watzlawick, 1990), interpersonal changes and modification in reinforcement schedules, etc. – *better* is better, *different* is different, and more of the same does not make a change.

---

was unmotivated and unhelpful – until she revealed that her mother had recently died and the plumber said his mother was dead also but that his father, a difficult man, was still living. "You miss them when they're gone no matter what they were like, I said." "How about your mother?" he wanted to know. "How old was she?" In that moment, they connect through their shared humanity. The man became helpful, and even returned to check the gas line heating the water tank. As he was leaving, he saw some old Polaroid photos and paused: "Oh, you'll want those," he said, "That's memories right there." It's not SST and all the social issues are not resolved, of course, but in the single encounter emotional connection opened a frontier.

7.   *Consider taking a time-out.* A break or pause during a session allows time to think, consult, focus, prepare, punctuate. Don't do all the work; if the client says "I dunno" the therapist can say "I dunno, either – let's sit and think about it for a while." Some training programs and clinics have (with the client's consent) observers behind a one-way mirror with call-in phones. One time when I was befuddled (it happens), I excused myself and went into the hall to implore a colleague, "What the hell should I do?" He calmed me down, reminded me of a similar case ("This sounds kind of like the case we talked about last week – except this is a woman and that was a man. What did you do then that helped?") and then gently directed me back into the therapy room. It was a "single session hall consultation"! (see Hoyt, 2017, p. 305)

8.   *Allow time for last-minute issues.* "Eleventh-hour" questions should be asked about "six o'clock," to allow time for inclusion or prioritization. It may be helpful to ask, "Before we talk about possible ways to deal with this problem is there anything else you think I need to know?" Unaddressed issues may impede a sense of the session being complete and satisfactory.

9.   *Give feedback.* Information should be provided that enhances the client's understanding and sense of self-mastery. If asked, I'm willing to provide a diagnosis (I might even pull the *DSM* off the shelf and ask the client to help me determine if they have "at least five of the following eight criteria," etc.) Saying, "You have a very active imagination, and sometimes you use it to think of scary, stressful things, but if you're interested we could talk about ways you could use your imagination to help you stay calm" (see Pelletier, 1977) is almost always more helpful than just saying "You have Generalized Anxiety Disorder." (Oh, G.A.D.!) Similarly, saying to someone who is getting exhausted from being a compulsive caregiver, "You're a very caring person. Would you be interested in talking about some ways you can be caring toward yourself? You know, the New Golden Rule: 'Do Unto Yourself As Well As You Do Unto Others'" will probably lead to a better outcome than just saying "You're co-dependent, you're enmeshed, and you have poor boundaries." In addition to (or part of) giving feedback, tasks or "homework" may be developed that will continue therapeutic work (see Figure 3.2 below).

10. *Leave the door open.* The decision to stop (or return) is usually best left to the client.

Stages of Change

"The readiness is all."
—Shakespeare (*Hamlet*, Act V, Scene II)

As James Prochaska (1999) has described it, clients may be at different stages of readiness.

> *Precontemplation* is the stage at which there is no intention to change behavior in the foreseeable future.
>
> *Contemplation* is the stage in which people are aware that a problem exists and are seriously thinking about overcoming it but have not yet made a commitment to take action.
>
> *Preparation* is a stage that combines intention and behavior criteria. Individuals in this stage are intending to take action immediately and report some small behavioral changes.
>
> *Action* is the stage that combines intention and behavior, experiences, and/or environment in order to overcome their problems.
>
> *Maintenance* is the stage in which people work to prevent relapse and consolidate the change. Stabilizing behavior change and avoiding relapse are the hallmarks.
>
> *Termination* is the stage in which there is zero temptation to engage in the problem behavior, and there is virtually 100 percent confidence (self-efficacy – Bandura, 1986) that one will not engage in the old behavior regardless of the situation.

Recognizing the client's stage of readiness will help to gauge which therapy strategies may be most efficacious for engendering change in an SST (Hoyt & Miller, 2000):

> *Precontemplation:* Suggest that the client "think about it" and provide information and education.
>
> *Contemplation:* Encourage thinking, recommend an observation task in which the client is asked to join with the client's lack of commitment to action with a 'Go slow' directive.
>
> *Preparation:* Offer treatment options, invite the client to choose from viable alternatives.
>
> *Action:* Amplify what works – get details of success and reinforce. Cheerlead, don't mislead.
>
> *Maintenance:* Support success, predict setbacks, make contingency plans. It is often better to speak of 'relapse management' rather than 'relapse prevention' – 'Since challenges may come up, how can you make it a small slip rather than an avalanche?'
>
> *Termination:* Wish well, say goodbye, leave an open door for possible return if needed.

The Temporal Structure of Sessions

In SST, each session is a stand-alone, one-off, potentially complete-unto-itself event. There is often a temporal structure to single sessions, with different issues and tasks associated with the different stages of a meeting. Figure 3.1 and the following discussion can serve as a general roadmap – although the art and craft of therapy is how one customizes to fit the particular client, therapist, and situation.

The course of each therapy session can be conceptualized as having five phases or stages: pretreatment, early, middle, late, and follow-through. They tend to be pyramidal or epigenetic – that is, they tend to occur in sequence and each flows from the preceding, so that successful work in one preconditions the next. The client elects therapy before forming an alliance; the alliance establishes the ground for defining goals; goal setting leads to focusing on specific change strategies, homework, relapse prevention, and leave-taking; and points toward continued growth and possible return to treatment.

There is often a microcosm-macrocosm parallelism in which the structure of each therapy session tends to mirror (or parallel) the overall course of a brief therapy (see Gustafson, 1986, p. 279; Hoyt, 2017, p. 213). Issues usually involved in the first portion of treatment are similar to those involved in the first portions of each session; the middle of treatment resembles the middle of each session; the issues that characterize the later portions of therapy tend also to characterize the later portions of each session. All of this comes together when the one session is the whole treatment: SST. As biologists might say, "Ontogeny recapitulates phylogeny – the development of the

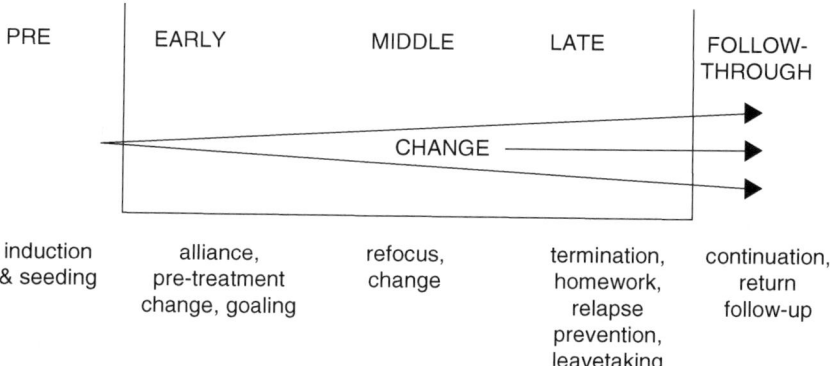

Figure 3.1 The Temporal Structure of SST

Source: ©M.F. Hoyt, 1995. Used with permission.

individual mirrors the development of the species"; crystallographers and chaos theorists may prefer to think about "fractals," never-ending patterns that are self-similar across different scales; poets may conceptualize the parallel as a kind of "synecdoche," in which a part is put forward to represent the whole.[4]

Useful Questions at Different Junctures

Michele Weiner-Davis (1993, p. 156) cogently wrote: "Since we cannot avoid leading, the question becomes, 'Where shall we lead our clients?'" Recognizing key questions often associated with different phases of an effective session can make treatment – be it SST or longer – more focused and efficient. As my colleagues Simon Budman, Steven Friedman, and I wrote in *The First Session in Brief Therapy* (1992), it is important to introduce novelty, since more of the same does not make a change. Describing a preferred future, using mental imagery and other techniques, can help the client to begin to have a glimpse of the possible, engendering hope and helping them to see that they can make a change.

> The novelty may come by seeing oneself differently, by practicing new ways of transacting with others, by experiencing unacknowledged feelings, by utilizing strengths and abilities that were previously overlooked. Whatever the means, [the single session] therapist looks for ways to start or amplify the clients' movement in the desired direction as soon as possible.
>
> (Hoyt, 1995, p. 289)

The right questions can guide attention toward strengths and solutions. The doors of therapeutic perception and possibility were opened wide by the recognition that we are actively constructing our mental realities rather than simply uncovering or coping with an objective "Truth" (Hoyt, 2017, p. 70). Good to remember that we are not just "taking history" but are "making history" (Hoyt, 2017, p. 95).

---

4   As William Blake (1806/1966) wrote:

>   To see a World in a Grain of Sand
>   And a Heaven in a Wild Flower
>   Hold Infinity is the palm of your hand
>   And Eternity in an hour.

But how is it
That this lives in thy mind? What seest thou else
In the dark backward and abysm of time?
> William Shakespeare, *The Tempest* (Act I, Scene 2, lines 48–50)

As Carlos Sluzki (1988, 1992, 1998; also see Friedman, 1993, 1996, 1997; Gergen, 1998; McNamee & Gergen, 1992; Tilden, Solem, Thuen, Loräs, Stokkebekk, & Whitaker, 2024) noted, constructivism is a way of thinking about therapy, not a specific school or approach. "Better-formed stories" appeal to those who consult us, are richer in connections between individuals and contexts, do not require self-perpetuating diagnostic labels, contain assumptions about evolution and change, progress and hope; and define the participants as active, competent, responsible, and reflexive.

From his narrative constructivist viewpoint, Don Meichenbaum (in Hoyt, 1996/2001e, p. 114; also see Hoyt, 2002; Meichenbaum 2012, 2023) said:

> My own approach is to remain much more phenomenologically oriented, using the client's metaphors. From my perspective, it is better to 'unpack' the client's metaphors rather than to impose the therapist's metaphors. By 'unpack,' I mean help the client to appreciate the adaptive features of how he or she has constructed reality in the past, but to also consider anew what is the impact, toll, and price of continuing to view the world in such a fashion – moreover, to consider in some detail what exactly can be done to change his or her 'construction,' as well as the ways he or she behaves. From this perspective, the client's altered narrative becomes the 'final common pathway' to behavioral change.

A myriad of helpful competence- and solution-identifying questions are provided in DeJong and Berg (1997), de Shazer et al. (2007), Ratner et al. (2012), Hoyt (2017), Dryden (2019b), Connie and Froerer (2023), and Murphy (2024), amongst others. Here is a sample, arrayed by when they might likely be asked in a therapy session (although they could be used whenever it seems appropriate). Imagine asking a client these guideline questions. Feel free to adapt (and adopt!) them; you may want to read them aloud or perhaps role-play asking them with a colleague.

Pre-Treatment. Change begins even before meeting the client – he/she/ they have decided there is a problem and would like assistance. Entering the client's worldview ("speak their language") builds the nascent therapeutic alliance. To help "hit the decks running," if you (or a triage screener) have an opportunity to speak with the client before meeting, here are some typical questions that could be asked, on the telephone or via the internet:

- What's the problem? *How* is the problem a problem – how is it affecting your life?
- Why have you called now (rather than earlier or later)? (Budman & Gurman, 1988)
- How do you see or understand the situation?
- What do you think will help? What skills and resources do you have that may be useful (Dryden, 2017)?
- How have you tried to solve the problem so far – how did that work?
- Please notice between now and when we meet, so that you can describe it to me, when the problem isn't so bad, what are you doing differently then? (de Shazer, 1985; Weiner-Davis et al., 1987; Weiner-Davis, 1995)

Early in the Session. When the client arrives in the office, questions such as these can be helpful to strengthen the alliance, establish a focus, find out about any developments since the client decided to seek therapy and to emphasize the client's initiative and accountability:

- Since we spoke [*or*, since you contacted the clinic], what have you noticed that may be a bit better or different? How did that happen? What did you do?
- When is the problem not a problem? When the problem isn't present (or isn't so bad), what is going on differently? ("exceptions," de Shazer, 1985, 1988). Carl Hammerschlag (1988, p. iv) noted: "Milton Erickson, that master hypnotherapist, understood that to begin a story by saying 'Remember when' was already to begin to place the audience into an altered state of consciousness – the very act of remembering is a kind of trance in itself." Asking someone to "remember when" also implies that there have been exceptions to be recalled or (re)discovered – the difference can be "put to work" (de Shazer, 1991b).
- What do you call the problem? What name do you have for it? (White & Epston, 1990)
- When (and how) does the problem influence you; and when (and how) do you influence it? (externalization and relative influence questioning, White & Epston, 1990)
- What's your idea or theory about what will bring about change? How would your life be better with these changes? (motivational interviewing, Miller & Rollnick, 1991; Miller, 2000)

- Suppose tonight, while you're sleeping, the problem gets worse – "how would your life be?" (the "Nightmare Question," Reuss, 1997) (*or:* "What would you need to do to make your problem worse?" – Fisch, Weakland, & Segal, 1982; Nardone & Watzlawick, 1990)
- If I told you that we were only going to meet once, what problem would you want to focus on solving at this point in time? (Haley, 1989) (*or:* "Given all the issues you've mentioned, which is the most important for us to focus on today?")
- What needs to happen here today so that when you leave you can feel this visit was worthwhile? (Hoyt & Berg, 1998/2000)
- What are you willing to change today? (Goulding & Goulding, 1979)
- Given all that you have been through, how have you managed to cope as well as you have? (solution-focused therapy coping/endurance question, de Shazer, 1988) *or* How have you all managed to keep things from getting worse? (de Shazer et al., 2007, p. 5)
- If we work hard and well together, what will be the first small indications that we are going in the right direction? (Miller, 1992)
- On a scale of 0–10, where is the problem now? Where would it need be for you to decide that you didn't need to continue coming here? (Berg & de Shazer, 1993; Vitry et al. 2024).
- Suppose tonight, while you're sleeping, a miracle happens, and the problem that led you here is resolved. When you awaken tomorrow, how will you first notice the miracle has happened? What will be the first sign that things are better? And the next? And the next? (the "Miracle Question," de Shazer, 1988)
- What other things will you be doing in the future that will tell you that you will no longer be needing our help? (Ziegler & Hoyt, 2023)
- What are your best hopes for today's meeting? (Shennan & Iveson, 2012; Iveson, George, & Ratner, 2014)
- How will your life be different if these hopes are realized? (Iveson, 2019)
- What do you know about yourself that lets you know you can achieve what you want? (Connie & Froerer, 2023)
- What are you already doing or have done in the past that might help bring these hopes to fruition? (Iveson, 2019)

In the Middle of the Session. As Nick Cummings put it, our contract with clients should be that we are available as long as they truly need us, and their contract should be to make us obsolete as soon as possible (Cummings & Sayama, 1995); and family therapists Salvador Minuchin and Michael Nichols (1998) advised that therapy may take place in the office, but change takes place at home. The purpose of therapy is not just to have a good therapist-client relationship; the therapeutic alliance should be the vehicle, not the destination. Application is key here: what is the client doing to make changes outside the consulting room? Ultimately, the purpose of therapy is for the client to handle and resolve their problems so that they no longer need therapy; done well, therapists talk themselves out of a job! Termination should be the goal.

Questions such as these can help to keep track of the client's goals and to make sure we're allied and going in the right direction. Possible refocusing can be directed by the client's responses:

- How did that work? What did you do to help it happen?
- Is this being helpful to you? What would make it more so?
- Are we working on what you want to work on?
- I might have missed something – what might that be?
- Do you have any questions you'd like to ask me?
- Would you like to pause and take a little break before we go on? (see Sharry et al. 2001)
- What hasn't been said that is important?
- Is there anything else that you feel I need to know in order to be helpful to you today?

Late in the Session. In SST (and brief therapy), ending is never far off: "termination is our frame" (Goldfield, 1998, p. 243). Termination – extracting the therapist from the successful equation (Gustafson, 1986) – becomes central. While we can recognize that termination in some ways may be a pseudo-event in that the work continues and formal treatment can be intermittently resumed, it is important to end well in order to maximize the likelihood that, while the therapy may be brief, the benefit may be long term.

Generally speaking, "The bigger the Hello, the bigger the Goodbye" – meaning the more connected the client and clinician become, the more likely will termination become a significant event; but if the SST work is relatively straightforward, termination may be relatively simple. As noted in Rosenbaum et al. (1990/1995, pp. 135–136), when concluding an SST, we may first ask the client if he or she feels that enough has been accomplished in the session to help him or her move on. If the answer is yes, we may ask for a description of what it was, to encourage lexical encoding, storage, and recall of a useful lesson. At other times, we may prefer to have the client leave with a more diffuse sense that "something" changed or will change soon. In all cases, we let clients know that we will remain available on an as-needed basis. We may encourage them, however, to take some time on their own to consolidate their gains.

If we stop after an important piece of work has been partially accomplished but before all of its ramifications are specifically spelled out, it is good to remember that we tend to process "unfinished business" (Perls, 1969) or incomplete tasks more than completed ones (Zeigarnik, 1938), so ending an SST in this fashion may help the client to get "unstuck" and allow the client to continue the work of the therapy on his or her own. The degree of closure appropriate to termination covers a wide range, and it is influenced by the extent to which the therapy was seeking resolution of some issue or attempting to open up new possibilities. Since some SST clients will in the future seek further therapy, it is important to structure the termination in such a way that a decision for more treatment will be seen by the client as an opportunity for further growth rather than an indicator of failure.

Dryden (2021, pp. 43–45) suggests encouraging the client to engage in a "reflect-digest-act-wait-decide" process in which the client takes time to absorb and use what has occurred in a single session before booking another meeting. In a more recent paper, Dryden (2023) has emphasized that SST/OAAT should not restrict clients to only one session nor to how often or soon they might return for another session. Clients should be allowed to return at their point of need/request without an arbitrary pause or mandatory hiatus. Indeed, if I saw an SST client for a session and they said, "Can I come back in two days for another meeting?" I'd likely say "Yes" and encourage them in the interim to think about what we had talked about and what they want to accomplish.

Application is key. Michael White (1992, p. 81) thus wrote: "It is not enough for a person to tell a new story about oneself, or to assert claims about oneself. Instead [...] it is the performance of these texts that is transformative of person's lives." It can be helpful for the client to have something to do post-session (which may be called *next steps* or *homework* or *practice opportunities* or *experiments*). The therapist can design and assign such activities, but it is usually better if the client suggests it and/or clinician and client collaboratively develop whatever will be next (rather than the therapist assigning it) in order to further empower the client and increase their buy-in (see Sharry et al., 2021). Dryden (2017, pp. 197–204) recommends, at the end of the face-to-face session, offering the client a summary of the session (and even a recording and transcript), tidying up loose ends, and securing their commitment toward implementing what they have learned. Other therapists, even if they may eschew strategic assignments, still encourage clients to carry on and apply what is helpful. Steve de Shazer (in Hoyt, 1996/2001, pp. 159–161) contended that once a therapist has identified exceptions to the problem:

You don't need strategies, or you don't need 'strategic maneuvers' *à la* Haley or Haley's interpretation of Erickson, or even the earlier MRI stuff. I found out that when we switched from problem solving to solution development, you just don't need to do that sort of thing. You don't need these fancy interventions. [...] It's no more effective than the simple things we are doing, maybe even less effective. Certainly they are far more work than what we're doing now. [...] I think that the compliments and the way we do the interview [...] will lead the clients to spontaneously reframe things for themselves. The only reframe that counts is if the client buys it. So the best ones are the ones they come up with.

Martin Söderquist (2023, p. 77) writes: "I prefer the words *idea, suggestion,* or *experiment* because they are more open, more generous and less forcing. I always tell the couple they are in the driver seat and it is their decision." Bobele and Slive (2014, p. 104) also wrote:

In the majority of sessions [...] there is the addition of a homework task or an idea that maintains the change begun by the therapy session. We have recently experimented with asking clients to use the break to design their own homework assignment or task that will assist them in taking the next step toward achieving their goals. [...] Sometimes there may be a rather elaborate task designed to address the current dilemma. Other times, the task may be as simple as an idea for client self-care.

These guideline questions suggest a number of issues to be considered, including goal attainment, homework/post-session tasks, relapse prevention, and leave-taking:

- Has this been helpful to you? How so?
- How might you recall some of the things we've discussed after the session?
- Which of the helpful things we've discussed do you think you should continue to do? How can you do this?
- To keep things going in the right direction, would you be willing to _____?
- What are you most likely to do with today's session?
- Who can be helpful to you in doing _____?
- What might interfere, and how can you prepare to deal with those challenges?

- What is the longest you can imagine handling things on your own?
- Do you know how to reach [me, the Clinic, emergency services] if/when you want to contact us?

Follow-Through. Everything may not be resolved by the end of the session, of course, but the client has learned or recalled some useful skills and has enhanced motivation. Benefit and change may continue after the meeting with the client. Here are some questions that could be asked in a follow-up questionnaire or call (see Talmon, 1990, pp. 127–128; also see Dryden, 2019b, pp. 247–250):

- How have you been doing in terms of the issues we discussed?
- On a scale from 0 to 10, where would you now rate the problem?
- How did you help that to happen?
- What do you recall about the session that was particularly helpful or harmful?
- Did you find the single session to be sufficient? If not, was treatment continued here or elsewhere?
- If you had any recommendations for improvement, what would they be?
- Would you like to wait and see how things go and call me as needed, or schedule an appointment now?

ARRIVALS AND DEPARTURES: SPECIAL ATTENTION TO BEGINNING AND ENDING AN SST

Aristotle said, "A good start is half the job." The negotiation of achievable goals is a major key to working efficaciously, whatever the length of treatment. It quickly and actively involves the client; engenders hope and energy by envisioning a better, obtainable future; and helps keep treatment brief by establishing a reachable endpoint. As Fisch (1994, p. 131) wrote:

> How long or short therapy is also depends on whether the therapist knows when to stop. It may seem trite to say, but if one has no idea of when something is done one runs the risk of going on interminably. Therapy, therefore, can be briefer if the therapist has some rather clear idea of what needs to occur to mark an endpoint of therapy.

Haley (1977, p. 9) describes the importance of framing a problem in such a way that it can be solved: "If therapy is to end properly, it must begin properly – by negotiating a solvable problem. [...] The act of therapy begins

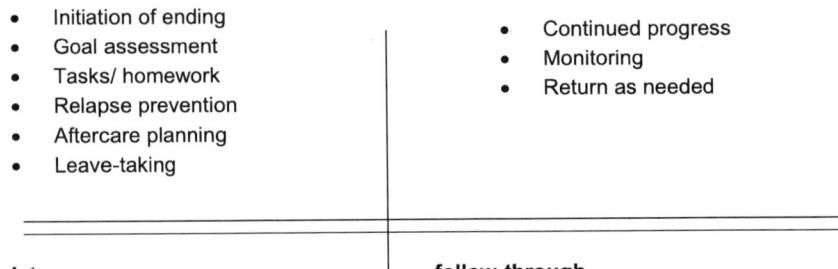

- Initiation of ending
- Goal assessment
- Tasks/ homework
- Relapse prevention
- Aftercare planning
- Leave-taking

- Continued progress
- Monitoring
- Return as needed

late

follow-through

Figure 3.2 The Ending Phase – Termination of a Session and a Treatment

Souce: ©M.F. Hoyt 1995. Used by agreement.

with the way the problem is examined." How we begin and how we finish can be especially important. Primacy effects set the tone and direction; recency effects promote application and follow-through (see Hoyt, 2017, pp. 153–176). Therapy should be brief by *design* not by *default* (Budman & Gurman, 1988). This is also what Bloom (1992, p. 3) meant by *planned*: "treatment that is intended to accomplish a set of therapeutic objectives within a sharply limited time frame."

Figure 3.2 shows some issues to consider when finishing an SST (see Hoyt, 2000b; Hoyt & Rosenbaum, 2018).

In SST (as in other therapies), everything may not be settled or completely resolved by the end of the session(s). The client may get "unstuck" and back "on track" (Walter & Peller, 1994) but what are her/his/their next steps? de Shazer (in Hoyt, 1996/2001a, p. 179) favored constructive minimalism: "Wittgenstein (1980, p. 77e) has some tremendous advice for all authors: 'Anything your reader can do for himself, leave to him.'" In their recent revision of SFBT, Elliott Connie and Adam Froerer (2023, especially pp. 228–238) worry that paying compliments, summarizing, and/or assigning homework or tasks actually may undercut clients' autonomy and agency.

In my experience, it can be helpful for the client to consider how they will apply what has happened and engage in post-session tasks that will reinforce, consolidate, and extend the work done during the session (see Carlson, 2000; Beaulieu, 2004; Dryden, 2021; Hoyt, 2017). Some tasks or post-session activities may seem obvious – relaxation is the opposite of stress and anxiety; communication is the opposite of isolation; deliberately making small errors is the opposite of rigid perfectionism. Uninvited advice is seldom welcome and even less often heeded, however, so rather than the therapist designing and assigning a task, it is usually best if the client is prompted to nominate what they think will be helpful (which might be increasing an already existing exception to the problem or by doing something new and different). As Blaise Pascal (1623–1662) said in his *Pensées*: "We are usually convinced more easily by reasons we have found ourselves than by those which have occurred to others."

Sometimes seemingly easy and benign tasks don't actually get done. There may be various reasons for this:

- The client was not really interested or does not believe complying will help.
- The client does not remember how to complete the task.
- Factors in the client's life make compliance difficult.

There are steps that can be taken to increase the likelihood that a task will actually get done:

- Be sure assignments contain specific details about desired behavior. Have client design (or co-design) task.
- Give direct skill training when necessary (e.g., relaxation training).
- Reward compliance – elicit positive responses of client and others – "How will you feel? Who else will be glad to hear about it?"
- Begin with homework that is likely to be successfully accomplished – the "foot in the door" technique.
- Develop a system that will remind the client of the assignment (e.g., written note take-aways, memory cues, other people).
- Have the client make a public commitment – "Will you do it?" To "anchor" their agreement (as they would say in Neurolinguistic Programming – Bandler & Grinder, 1979), shake their hand or nod and smile approvingly when they say "Yes."
- The client should believe in the value of the assignment for treating his or her problem – "Does that make sense?" As mentioned above, have the client do something they've done before and/or have the client help develop the task, so that it will be practical and fit within the context of their real life.
- Use cognitive rehearsal strategies – prepare for stressors, practice confronting stressors, have patient reward self for completing homework (see Meichenbaum 1985, 2012). "What if it rains the day you plan to go on the picnic with your partner – then what will you do instead to have time together?"
- Anticipate and reduce the negative effects of a task – "It may be difficult and Joe/Jane may not like it, but it will be worth it to feel better – right?"

Dryden (2017, 2021) rightly emphasizes the importance of encouraging clients to make the effort and to tolerate some adversity as they make changes: "No pain, no gain."

- Ask them to let you know when they do the task (to heighten accountability and to promote internalization of the therapeutic alliance and the gains achieved in an SST). Many times I've come into my office in the morning to find my telephone message light flashing: "Hi Doctor. I just wanted to let you know that last night I went to a meeting [or "I used that visualization exercise we discussed" or "I started to get really angry but then remembered what we talked about" or "…."]. I'm okay. I'll call back if I need to come in."

To Follow Up, or Not to Follow Up? From the Italian Center for Single Session Therapy, Cannistrà (2018/2021, p. 111) writes:

> Although follow-up is often seen as the prerogative of a research context, it plays an essential role in our SST model. But we must be clear that this is also part of its modular approach and professionals and facilities are therefore free to choose whether to include it. […] In our work, telephone follow-ups usually last 10–15 minutes max. We ask how the previous three weeks have gone, if the client thinks there has been an improvement, and if he or she thinks that things are going well, or needs another session. Here too we are very flexible: the door can be left completely open, telling individuals to call if and when they want, about the same problem or others; or, if we evaluate together that the client is uncertain (for example, someone feels better, but is not sure about keeping up the results), we can suggest an appointment to check at a somewhat distant date (for instance, in another three weeks). Whatever happens, the important thing is to always leave the door open.

Asking for feedback can be useful and instructive, and you don't want to unnecessarily abnegate the therapeutic relationship and sense of continuity of care – but as Slive and Bobele (2018, pp. 35–36; also see Bobele & Slive, 2021 p. 58) note in their discussion of walk-in OAAT/SST, you also don't want to undermine the client by implying that you're asking for follow-up because you're not confident about the client's decision to stop after the one session. (Situations involving high-risk may require follow-up contact.) Talmon (1990, p. 115) notes:

Whether a therapist considers a single session as potentially valuable and sufficient therapy or as a dropout failure is a reflection of that therapist's attitude toward the phenomenon of SST in general. SST may very well threaten some therapists' egos, their theoretical orientation, and, last but not least, their pocketbooks. Termination in therapy is traditionally explored in the psychotherapy literature as primarily the client's problem (fears of abandonment, independent-dependent conflict, transference and separation anxieties, and so on). Yet single-session encounters present a difficult challenge to therapists: they are left in the dark as to whether the patient rejected their advice or invitation for further therapy, they are unable to get rewarding feedback about how useful or helpful they were to the patient, and they receive very little or no monetary reward for their efforts.

Additional logistical and practical factors may also play a role. Slive and Bobele (2018, p. 36) observe:

> There are other issues to be considered. We have limited staffing, which would make it inordinately difficult to attempt follow-up with the high volume of cases seen. We have also found that communicating with clients by telephone is extremely difficult – they may call us for information and to schedule appointments, but calling them back to confirm appointments, to reschedule appointments, etc. is usually met with either a non-answer or a voicemail greeting; messages are rarely returned. Another factor is that a model of service delivery with a built-in follow-up, we think, could encourage therapists to conduct sessions knowing that loose ends could be resolved on follow-up; our model, instead, encourages therapists to approach each session as if it were the *last* opportunity that the therapist(s) will have to work with the client. Clinicians and researchers may be curious about what happens after clients leave a session, but we know of no research demonstrating better outcomes for clients if there is a follow-up contact. So, it is hard to justify the added cost.[5]

---

5 Of course, as Carl Sagan (Feres & Feres, 2023) said, "Absence of evidence is not evidence of absence." Some SST clinicians and services use pre-session preparatory and/or after-therapy follow-up contacts, whereas others do not. Whether such contacts may produce better outcomes (and if so, how and for whom?) are empirical questions. Researchers, start your engines!

SST in a Nutshell

The basics of SST are working in a collaborative and culturally appropriate way:

1. Plan for one visit ("one-at-a-time")
2. Identify the client's goal for the session (which may involve hearing their "problem" or "complaint" and helping them recognize that something different needs to be done to get a different result)
3. Look for strengths and abilities that can be used to make a desired change
4. Encourage application in problematic situation, and
5. Leave the door open for possible follow-up.

Appendix B provides short checklists that can be used to guide Pre-Session Contact, Beginning the Session, and Closing the Session.

Access Options: SST/OAAT by Appointment or by Walk-In

A prospective client might sign up in advance for a by-appointment SST/OAAT session, as when someone calls a counseling agency that advertises providing SST or contacts a university counseling center that explicitly lists SST/OAAT as an option. The service website may even describe what problems are most likely and less likely to benefit from an SST appointment, such as:

Most likely for SST:

- Life transitions, decision making, relationship challenges, time management, stress and anxiety, worries about a friend or loved one, immediate concerns that you are ready to tackle with a plan of action; as well as couple/family issues with communication, parenting challenges, and financial decisions.

Not recommended for SST:

- Crisis interventions and emergencies, chronic mental-health problems, prolonged self-exploration.

Or the client may not be sure what length of therapy they want or need so they make a general intake appointment and then respond affirmatively when told

Some people are able to get what they need in one session. Let's see how it goes and at the end of the meeting we can evaluate whether one session has been enough for now or if you'd like to make another appointment.

A prospective client may also be asked to visit a website or otherwise read about a problem and then decide if they want to make an appointment; getting such information may be all they want/need at a particular moment (see Cornish, 2020).

Another valuable SST portal is via drop-in/walk-in (or, with modern technology, possibly via click-in or call-in). As noted earlier, the walk-in SST option was developed and promulgated at the Eastside Family Centre (EFC) in Calgary, Canada, and elsewhere (see Slive, MacLaurin, Oaklander, & Amundson, 1995; Slive & Bobele, 2011; Stewart et al., 2018; McElheran, 2021, in press). As Slive, McElheran, and Lawson (2008, p. 6) wrote:

> Developed [...] as a result of community demands for greater accessibility to mental-health services, walk-in therapy enables clients to meet with a mental-health professional as their moment of choosing. There is no red tape, no triage, no intake process, no wait list, and no wait. There is no formal assessment, no formal diagnostic process, just one hour of therapy focused on clients' stated wants. [...] Also, with walk-in therapy there are no missed appointments or cancellations, thereby increasing efficiency.

Although walk-ins do not allow time for elaborate pre-session preparations, the walk-in option maximizes the convenience and likelihood of providing services at what Dryden (2019a; also see Bundy, 2022) has called the *point of need* (rather than the *point of availability*). It fits well with other "walk-in" services that people have come to expect and appreciate, including banking, hairdressers, restaurants, tax preparers, "no wait" medical offices, etc. Walk-ins may be especially attractive at training centers and clinics with salaried staff (and volunteers) who can be waiting and available for persons who arrive without an appointment, whereas walk-ins may be more difficult to arrange for professionals in independent private practice who manage their own schedules.

There are many advantages to walk-ins for increasing access to services – and walk-in clinics are becoming more and more popular with research evidence supporting their utility. Slive and Bobele (2018) have highlighted three reasons that walk-in services "make perfect sense":

- *They seize the moment*, allowing clients to easily meet with a clinician at times of high motivation for change
- *They are effective*, as demonstrated by a growing body of research evidence (e.g., Miller & Slive, 2004; Miller, 2008; Slive & Bobele, 2011, in press; also see Hymmen et al., 2013; Harper-Jaques & Foucault, 2014; see Appendix A)
- *They are efficient*, reducing/eliminating waiting lists and avoiding client use of more expensive services such as emergency rooms.

Bobele and Slive (2021, in press; Slive & Bobele, 2019a, 2019b) have also identified and addressed common worries that some providers and clinic managers may have about adding the walk-in option to their services. They include:

- Will we be overwhelmed?
- How do you manage risk when clients just walk in?
- What about paperwork?
- If they just walk in, is there no pre-assessment?
- Is it ethical to not routinely follow-up after walk-in sessions?
- Can just anybody walk in?
- What if clients want something that we don't provide?
- What about clients who may be in therapy elsewhere?
- What if they are seeking an ongoing series of sessions?
- Do clients use a walk-in service as ongoing therapy?
- Are walk-in services suitable for minority and marginalized populations?
- What about structure, training, and support for new walk-in services?

While these are legitimate concerns, there are reasonable answers. Slive and Bobele note that many years of experience have shown that walk-ins do not increase risks or overwhelm services. Indeed, just the opposite. The walk-in option maximizes access to services, and clients (and society) greatly benefit. Bobele and Slive (2021, p. 57) observe the frequent concern clinicians express about possibly "missing something" in a single session, including potential risk factors. They note that the need for possible further risk assessment can be identified with one item in a client's intake materials, such as "Do you now, or have you had, any fears that you (or your child, or anyone with you) is at risk of harm to themselves, others, or pets?" Along related lines, Paul Denborough, a psychiatrist in Melbourne, Australia, familiar with SST, remarked (https://events.bouverie.org.au/sst):

It's actually the perfect model to deal with risk – Single Session – because you see people quickly. You get the whole social network and family around them, and you try and fix the problem as soon as possible. You couldn't get a better way to manage risk, in my opinion.

SST (by walk-in or by-appointment) is not a panacea, of course, and in general more mental-health resources are needed. However, as my colleagues and I wrote elsewhere (Hoyt, Young, & Rycroft, 2021, p. 340):

> This concern [about SST/OAAT clients being at risk] would seem to be based on a misunderstanding: a view of a single session approach being limited to a one-only session with no allowance for identifying urgent or emergency risks, incorporating other resources, offering and planning follow-up, or referral to emergency services, etc. In single session practice, risk is managed by responding explicitly to the client's main or immediate concerns and is addressed in the same way as in any ongoing work (e.g., assessment; safety plan; support; additional services, including hospitalization if needed). Further, we would contend that making services more accessible and responsive is a more ethical approach than asking vulnerable and at-risk clients to fall back on their own resources and/or languish on a waitlist.

As Single Session/OAAT thinking and practice expands, we can expect and should welcome both more walk-in and more by-appointment SST services.

SST Examples from the Literature: Methods and Models

4

Here, we'll consider a mosaic of SST examples from the literature involving individuals, couples, and families and then in the next chapter consider a few SST examples from my own experience. The range of SST practices and possibilities is intended to be suggestive, not definitive or exhaustive, providing a plethora of theories, models, strategies, tactics, and language choices. Case examples are offered, sometimes with excerpts in the original authors' own words, to encourage learning from leading SST practitioners. Many approaches are illustrated, evidencing both the extensive clinical foundation of SST and presenting a wide array of options that may help answer for different readers the question, "What would be most useful with this client and this therapist in this situation?"

SST is an OAAT delivery approach, not limited to one theoretical orientation. Hence, it is good to keep in mind:

> The search [is] for a conceptualization that would allow a viable and parsimonious solution. The therapist needs to be versatile, innovative, and pragmatic, asking: 'What would help this [client] today?' [Clients] may need to begin a process or complete a process; they may need to take hold or to let go; they may need reassurance or confrontation; they may need to look at something deeply or to shift perspective. [...] Nothing works all the time, but what might work this time?
>
> (Hoyt, Rosenbaum, & Talmon, 1992, p. 63)

DOI: 10.4324/9781003468547-4

As will be seen, generally speaking "different [SST] therapists use their expertise primarily to help clients better use their own expertise" (Hoyt, Bobele, Slive, Young, & Talmon, 2018b, p. 15). When combined, "The expertise of the therapist, when allied with the expertise of the client, can be a potent force" (Dryden, 2020, p. 283).

Clinicians in SST usually function more as gardeners rather than mechanics, attempting to nurture and bring forth what is helpful rather than conceptualizing therapy in terms of tinkering with and trying to fix something that is broken. We endeavor to provide useful information and support. Sometimes we're cheerleaders, or witnesses and guides, or function like a theater director evoking a performance. Sometimes our role is similar to that of a midwife, who attends the process and provides a helping hand in case anything gets temporarily stuck. Occasionally, we may even serve as a kind of protector or lifeguard, catching people and saving them from potential hazards, assisting them to resolve problems without encouraging them to feel dependent or incompetent.

In considering potential SST methods, be versatile and pragmatic. One size doesn't fit all. Be selective and use what would likely be helpful with a particular client. Theory or understanding guides us to what we do (see Marrow, 1977), but we should hold our theories lightly. Too much theory can become a hindrance in the living moment of clinical practice (Whitaker, 1976/1982). In *The Name of the Rose*, Umberto Eco (1980/1983; quoted in Iveson, 1990, pp. 13–14) has the protagonist advise:

> The order that our mind imagines is like a net, or like a ladder, built to attain something. But afterwards, you must throw the ladder away, because you discover that, even if it was useful, it was meaningless [....] The only truths that are useful are instruments to be thrown away.

The cases presented here involve different theoretical orientations and techniques and all occurred within the framework of a planned or deliberate single session. (There are also more examples in Chapters 5 and 6.) Regardless of the specific theoretical approach, all planned SSTs tend to share essential features:

• Expectation of one session
• Identification of the client's goal for the session
• Emphasis on strengths and abilities that can be used to make a desired change
• Encouragement of application in problematic situation, and
• Leaving the door open for possible return and/or follow-up.

After each case presentation, some questions are provided to prompt reflection on possible lessons. Readers are encouraged to consult the original reports and to consider ways that they might apply some of the ideas and methods with their own clients.

A Potpourri of SST/OAAT Examples from the Literature

- Moshe Talmon (1990), in the first pages of *Single Session Therapy: Maximizing the Most of the First (and Often Only) Therapeutic Encounter*, recounts a follow-up call with a mother one year after she had an SST seeking help for feelings of being overwhelmed by having to deal with two small children. Note that when she reported she was taking better care of both herself and the children, the therapist responded by emphasizing her role in their alliance and her resourcefulness in the improvement (pp. 1–3):

> Thank you so much for your input. It is very valuable for me, and I am certainly happy for you. As a therapist I feel it is mostly you who deserve the credit for the changes. After all, it is you who decided that you had had enough and needed to do something about it. It is you who knew your kids so well and were able to communicate clearly to me about it, so that I could come up with a useful suggestion. Last, but not least, you have translated what I said in such a nice and effective manner, so that you and actually your entire family could benefit from your action.

In another case, when the therapist receives a referral from a pediatrician and contacts the family, he introduces himself as someone who helps families solve their problems (not as someone who solves the problems himself):

> 'I was asked to see you since I am an expert in helping children and families solve problems.' (p. 22) [He also asked the mother (p. 23), showing respect for her opinion:] 'What seems to be the problem in school?'

In the introduction to his 1993 follow-up book, *Single Session Solutions: A Guide to Practical, Effective, and Affordable Therapy*, Talmon (pp. 1–4) describes the single session therapy of "Jack," a man who sought psychological help because of the unrelenting guilt he was feeling after an automobile accident in which his wife was seriously injured. After listening attentively to his story,

I said, 'You are clearly depressed. You are feeling this way because you are a very caring, loving, and responsible husband and father. Your depression is your way of expressing to your family your regrets and sorrow for causing the accident.'

I paused and then continued:

Your coming here today to see me is not only the right step at the right time, but also a wise and courageous step: facing your own feelings and going to a psychologist about it. It is a difficult step for anyone to take. […]

'Now,' it seems to me that you are ready to recognize that none of us, including you, is perfect. Accidents, even very bad ones, happen to all of us at one time or another. Now that you have taken full responsibility for causing the accident you are ready today to go back to your regular self: being a responsible father and husband Now, you can also begin to see the other side of the coin: The accident made you recognize how grateful you are to have Kirsten and yourself alive, and bless your kids for being so full of life and love. I am sure you want to find a renewed way to show them your positive feelings.

As Talmon comments (p. 4) in discussing the case:

Jack was seen for single-session therapy (SST). The art of therapy, in this case, was to facilitate change that can lead to a practical and relatively immediate solution. I reframed the depression as an act of love and caring, thus removing the self-perpetuating guilt and shame, and then formed an avenue to a solution by showing how this 'act of care and love' could be expressed differently.

Talmon (1993, p. 73) notes: "These concepts represent an alternative to the traditional model in psychiatry and psychotherapy: psychohealth replacing psychopathology, solutions replacing problems, and partnership replacing patronization, domination, and hierarchy." He describes various cases and advises readers (1993, p. 112):

If you feel stuck and overwhelmed, you are probably overlooking certain elements that may reveal a possible alternative role in the story. You may want to create a different emphasis. Review events and relationships in order to include, exclude, or conclude differently.

Reflection question: How might you encourage the client to refocus their story to create or uncover healthier understandings and pathways?

_____
_____
_____
_____
_____
_____
_____
_____

- Bob Rosenbaum (1993) reported a successful 90-minute SST that involved a woman who sought hypnosis to help her with weight loss. As he noted (p. 109),

> Although strategic therapy meets clients at their view of the world and pays close attention to the exact language clients use in describing their complaints in order to stay close to the clients' immediate experience, this does not mean that strategic therapists take all clients' presenting problems at face value. Frequently, resolving the chief complaint involves exploring a complex web of interpersonal relationships and even [...] the intrapsychic meaning the problems holds for the client.

As the session opens, the therapist rapidly creates an opportunity to strengthen the therapeutic alliance and increase the client's motivation (p. 111):

> Before we start, I just wanted to mention to you that some colleagues and I have been doing some research, and we found out that a lot of people get better coming in just for a single visit. Now, I don't know if we can solve your problems in one visit, and certainly if we need to meet more, I'll be glad to schedule as many visits as it takes. But I wanted to let you know that if you want to work on solving your problem today, I'm willing to work hard on this if you are. Would you like that?

She assents. They then spend some time exploring her interests, abilities, and challenges, including that her mother has always been critical and fault-finding. The client mentions (p. 15) that "I have always had the weight of being an ideal child." She has a brother who is a drug addict, "and I have always been the one to get the good grades. I have never been a problem child. The only problem that I have had is being overweight."

Rosenbaum notes:

> This is a crucial statement. It states the problem in one sentence, and also offers an avenue to its solution. It therefore can function as a 'pivot chord,' a psychological space where a solution can emerge from what appears to be a problem.

The session progresses, Rosenbaum telling the patient:

> I think that there are a few things we can work on together that would be helpful for you, and hypnosis is one of them, and we can do that today, but I think for the hypnosis to work, there are going to be a few other things that you are going to have to do in terms of the dieting. Just as you know that hypnosis won't work without dieting, right. Well, dieting won't work without doing a few other things. Okay. I don't want to treat you with hypnosis now unless we can get an agreement to do these other things.

As Rosenbaum comments to the reader (1993, p. 119):

> This is an 'anticipation' technique in which the 'cure' precedes the treatment technique. It is rather like syncopation in music. Getting the client to agree to this technique will essentially solve the problem before any 'treatment' (i.e., hypnosis) is administered since it will indicate that the client had already made a fundamental change in attitude.

He gets the patient to make a commitment to resume her singing and tap dancing. Regarding her dieting, he says to her (p. 123) "That's a different matter" – which he notes is "Again, an indirect suggestion that the client's task is to find a way to be true to herself – i.e., be more autonomous." A six-month follow-up by a research colleague[1] indicated success:

---

1   In a research study, whether of SSTs or other therapies, follow-ups are usually done by someone other than the therapist to reduce the influence of "demand characteristic" (Orne, 1969) artifacts such as liking or not liking the therapist; whereas in general practice, it may be preferable to have

the patient had lost weight and maintained the loss, and she attributed the success to herself, not to the therapy. "When asked what was most helpful, she mentioned "relaxation" but said (p. 126) what was particularly helpful was "The insight. Realizing that my attempts to please my mother and her expectations of me put a heavy weight on me. [...] I decided to go back to school again and in this way to become myself again. The rest fell into place relatively easily, because I was able to stand up behind my own decisions."

In another case report, Rosenbaum (in Rosenbaum, Hoyt, & Talmon, 1990/1995, pp. 117–118) described an SST with a woman who, when asked what she wanted to accomplish, began the session by handing him a 10-page single-spaced typed narrative of her early life and current unhappiness. She obsessed back and forth about various issues and his repeated attempts to establish a session focus were unsuccessful. Then:

> The therapist noticed the patient wore a pretty crystal on a necklace, and the patient described how she used crystals for meditation. She pulled out a variety of crystals from her purse. The therapist decided to use hypnosis to indirectly further treatment goals (Wolberg, 1980) and had the patient choose two crystals 'of differing character' and hold one in each hand. A trance was induced by having her focus on the different sensations in each hand, where one crystal 'could be thought of as hard, but ordinary, common sense' while the other 'feels like it gives brilliance, healing, and comfort.' The patient was then asked to combine the two inside herself; she then reported strong sensations of strength and energy with accompanying imagery. She was then given suggestions that she would be able to use this experience in the near future, together with posthypnotic cues for regaining the sensations when needed. [...] On follow-up she was markedly less depressed, was less conflicted about her job, and had written some new children's stories she was attempting to get illustrated and published.

Rosenbaum's recent SST work has focused on behavioral medicine. In a case report (personal communication, 2023), he wrote:

> Another single session case involved a referral from the neurology clinic of a 30 year-old man who was suffering multiple complex

---

the therapist do the follow-up to maintain continuity of care and to promote internalization of the positive therapeutic relationship.

partial seizures every day. [...] It's a well-established fact that anxiety lowers seizure thresholds. For people with epilepsy, the more anxious they are, the more likely they are to have seizures. A common behavioral treatment for seizures is to teach patients relaxation techniques. In this case, however, the client's wife held more anxiety than the client.

When I pointed out to the couple how her anxiety exacerbated his seizures and his seizures exacerbated her anxiety, they readily agreed. Each acknowledged their role in the vicious cycle. They knew relaxation methods but had found they couldn't use them effectively. How could he relax when she was hovering? He'd asked her to give him more space. His wife felt badly about her hovering, but how could she back off while she feared he'd lose control during a seizure and harm himself?

I empathized and validated their experience. I acknowledged it wouldn't work for either of them to just tell themselves to relax. I suggested instead they each needed to help the other person by giving their partner relaxation *challenges*. Specifically, I suggested they arrange for the husband to go into a separate room several times a day to practice his relaxation – and suggested to the wife that she interrupt him unexpectedly, so he could learn how to stay calm even while she intruded.

Meanwhile, I suggested to the husband that in addition to whatever seizures occurred naturally, three times a day he should *pretend* to have seizures. That would give the wife a chance to say to herself 'Maybe I don't have to worry about this one,' to pause, practice her relaxation by taking a few breaths, and asking herself whether there really any imminent danger, regardless of whether or not the seizure was a pretend one. I suggested they set aside some time at the end of each day to brief each other on what they experienced – and how successful the wife had been on guessing which was a real seizure, and how successful the husband had been in teasing his wife by pretending. (Incidentally, most patients with epilepsy in fact experience a mixture of physiological and function-psychological seizures.)

As soon as they started doing this, the seizure frequency decreased to one seizure every few days. At this point, the neurologist was able to institute an effective medication regimen.

The therapy process was able to avoid getting caught in 'is' or 'is not.' We are not who we think we are, and our therapies are not what we think they are. Applying the same logic to SST, we realize single session therapies are not defined according to whether they are, or are not, confined to one session.

In 1982, Bob wrote (Rosenbaum, 1982, p. 89):

We also see now that ultimately, to the extent that paradoxical interventions invoke an experience that allows a patient to give up the hubris of having a reified, constant conception of himself and to permit himself to be consistently inconsistent, to that extent the patient can give up his symptoms. We are faced with a situation, then, in which it is the very experience of the self as empty, as lacking a solid core, that leads to a wider, stronger, healthier experience of the self. That is the paradox of paradox.[2]

Rosenbaum's multifaceted understanding of psychotherapy is informed by a variety of therapy orientations as well as by his long-time study of Zen Buddhism (e.g., see Rosenbaum, 1999, 2013, 2022, in press). A number of his quotable quotes speak to the essence of SST:

✓ "My desire is not to see everyone for one session; my desire is to see everyone for one full moment, as long as that takes" (from Hoyt, Rosenbaum, & Talmon, 1992, p. 80).

✓ "Psychotherapy is not long or short; to view it this way sets up a false dichotomy. Psychotherapy instead depends on 'good moments' where something profound shifts for a client. All the rest is preparation and consolidation." [...] Because we feel psychotherapy needs to focus more on these critical incidents of change, we no longer talk of 'single-session therapy' but prefer, instead, to examine 'therapy moment by moment'" (Rosenbaum, 2008, p. 8).

✓ "Therapy, like life, does not 'take' time because time is not a dimension we exist 'in.' We are time, and time is us [...] Nothing is ever finished, but everything is always complete" (Rosenbaum, 2014, pp. 48–50).

---

2   *Paradox* is a logically self-contradictory statement, situation, or action; it simultaneously gets you coming, going, and where you're at. Poet and critic Tony Hoagland (2014, p. 171) refers to "Paradox, cross-eyed cousin to logic." It baffles itself and requires an "epistemological leap" (Rosenbaum 1982) to escape. For more on the use of paradox in psychotherapy, see Palazzoli et al. (1978), Weeks and L'Abate (1982), and Loriedo and Vella (1992).

Reflection questions: (1) If not now, when? (2) How can you disrupt (or therapeutically utilize) a maladaptive interpersonal pattern?

_____

_____

_____

_____

_____

_____

_____

_____

- Pam Rycroft and Jeff Young (2021), illustrating how they translate single session thinking into practice, give an account of the case of "Georgie and Anne," a couple who sought an appointment to discuss their concerns regarding their 14-year-old son. During an angry outburst, he had threatened his younger brother with a knife. The parents wondered whether they had responded appropriately and/or whether their son needed psychiatric evaluation. After completing an intake questionnaire and having a brief telephone contact, they were then seen in session with the son. Careful attention was paid to connecting with all the participants, to complimenting Georgie and Anne for their concern, and to recognizing the son's strengths and not just his temper. To keep things focused on the search for solutions (Context of Competence), at one point the therapist remarked: "Given that we have about 20 minutes left [...] I'm wondering what hasn't been said – or asked – at this point?" The son had talked things out with his brother. He acknowledged his role in the altercation, was remorseful, and pledged to do better. Both Georgie and Anne felt reassured and validated, both in their concern and also in their parenting. Further discussion revealed no indication for additional psychiatric evaluation or treatment. They agreed to a phone follow-up in two weeks and to recontact the therapist sooner if needed. At follow-up, the family reported that at home they had talked more about the incident and the session. They were doing well, did not feel a need for another session, and expressed appreciation for the open-door invitation to return if/when appropriate.

Reflection question: What would indicate that one session has been sufficient or the need for additional sessions?

_____

_____

_____

_____

_____

_____

_____

- Jeff Young (2024), in *No Bullshit Therapy: How to Engage People Who Don't Want to Work with You*, recognizes the potentially daunting challenge of clients who are reluctant and resistant, especially those who can be described as "therapy-haters." He presents (p. 6) four NBT Clinical Guidelines designed to create contexts for working with mutual honesty and directness:

  1. Establish a mandate / agreement
  2. Marry honesty and directness with warmth and care
  3. Be upfront about constraints
  4. Avoid jargon.

He then goes on to illustrate with several examples how an SST / OAAT approach, which avoids obfuscating language and "beating around the bush," can be especially useful when working with such "difficult" and "resistant" people (pp. 76–77; italics in original):

> The techniques of Single Session Therapy provide useful guidance on how to make overt client and worker goals for the encounter. Gentle business engagement adds power and purpose to social engagement: *What brought you here today? How can I be most helpful to you today? What would you like to walk away with at the end of the session?* The techniques and questions of Single Session Therapy, derived from thinking that if this session is the last, what should I ask, explore, share, and do, helps to create a culture of directness. When both client and therapist consider that each session maybe the last, there is a natural tendency to *cut to the chase*. And the single session structure provides an obvious

boundary which provides safety; essentially the framework *this could be our last session* – so let's make the most of it allows clients to determine how deeply to go and how quickly to cut to the chase.

Reflection question: What might signal that a client would prefer a very direct, "No B.S" approach?

_____

_____

_____

_____

_____

_____

_____

_____

_____

• Brendan O'Hanlon and Naomi Rottem (2021; also see Le Gros, Wyder, & Brunelli, 2018; Fleming, 2021; Fuzzard, 2021; Renkin, Alexander, & Wyder, 2021; McDonald, Hickey, & Wyder, 2021; von Doussa, Tsorlinis, Cordukes, Beauchamp, & McIntosh, 2021) describe Single Session Family Consultation (SSFC), a model of brief family engagement and inclusion developed at The Bouverie Centre (Melbourne), in which an individual's ongoing care is supplemented by one to three sessions of a practitioner meeting with the client and the entire family to collaboratively respond to family-identified concerns and to clarify how the family will be involved in the individual's continuing care. The practitioner could be the client's regular therapist or a different individual.

Combining principles of family consultation (FC) and SST, SSFC involves three stages: *convening, conducting,* and *following-up*. The client can decide who will attend the consultation session(s) and what topics will (and will not) be discussed. As O'Hanlon and Rottem (p. 69) note, much of the process of the consultation session is informed by single session thinking:

✓ Family members are invited to prioritize issues that they want to address

✓ The practitioner checks in during the session about whether the current focus or the experience of the session is helpful

✓ An awareness of available time is encouraged to maximize the value of the session

✓ The practitioner is transparent in their process of conducting the session and in sharing reflections of the family's issues and dilemmas.

Reflection questions: What would tell you that a SSFC would be helpful? How might you introduce it to a client?

_____

_____

_____

_____

_____

_____

_____

• Arnie Slive and Monte Bobele (2011, pp. 37–63), Bobele and Slive (2014, pp. 101–105), and Bobele et al. (2018, p. 222) highlight their structure/agenda for a walk-in SST session:

1. Pre-session. Reviewing intake forms, preliminary planning
2. The session. Joining and establishing an alliance, defining the problem, and goal setting
3. Consultation break. Reviewing clients' strengths and resources, developing a plan, homework if appropriate
4. Closing. Strengths-based feedback. Assessing outcome of session. Next steps.
5. Debriefing. Reviewing with walk-in team what went well, what was learned, note writing.

As Cannistrà and Piccirilli (2021, p. 84) note, Slive and Bobele's model provides a clear operational structure, making it more easily transmissible for individuals and facilities seeking to implement it within a walk-in context.

Slive and Bobele (2012, p. 30) write:

Our minimal goals in walk-in therapy are for the clients to leave the session with a sense of emotional relief and increased hope. For one client, a positive outcome may be as straightforward as knowing that someone has heard their story. For another client, it could be a new way of thinking about a problem – the beginning of a new story. The new way of thinking about a problem may, in another instance, involve deciding that this is not a problem after all. Another client may leave the session with a specific task, a new way of approaching a troubling issue. Or a client may leave with ideas about where to get further help.

and (pp. 30–31):

> We begin each session assuming that it will comprise the whole therapy [...] We prefer to think of walk-in therapy as a consultation process in which the therapist offers ideas (many of which may have come from the client), and the client decides whether to accept them, reject them, or put them on hold. A consultation stance helps therapists to resist the temptation to take responsibility for client change. We believe that the clients are their own greatest resource. Clients are in the best position to evaluate the ideas generated during the session. Our job is to create a context that enables clients to discover those resources and teach us how to be their guide.

Slive and Bobele (2012) present a typical walk-case SST case. A couple, "Manny and Vera," came to the Community Counseling Service, a training clinic operated by Our Lady of the Lake University in San Antonio, Texas, that uses a team-based live supervision model. Some representative therapist comments:

- ✓ "You've come for what we call our walk-in service. You can come as you have today; you didn't need an appointment. If you want at some point in the future, you could come back in the same way. Some people find that one session works for them. You know, they get what they want from it and leave, and that's that. Some people decide they want to walk in again. Some people decide they'd like to make an appointment and see somebody here. When we get to the end, we can talk about that. So what are you hoping for today in coming here?"
- ✓ "And how did you guys come to the decision to come today to talk about those things?"
- ✓ "So if you were to begin to feel a little bit more hopeful, Manny, what might Vera see that would be a sign to her that you were more hopeful? What would she see?"
- ✓ "So that would be a big change."

✓ "And how would you know? Like what might he do that would tell you he's taken a step in that direction of showing you"

✓ "And, Manny, we also know that when you set your mind to get good at something, that you do it. You gave us a number of examples of things that you really have decided you were going to learn, and you just did it."

✓ "You both talked about Manny being more responsible in his work life. Manny, you've impressed all of us as somebody who, if you decided that you were going to figure out how to do that, it would be hard and it would take time, but you would do it. You would do it, because you've done it before. The best sign that you're going to do something in the future is if you've done it before."

Slive and Bobele (2012, pp. 35–36) concluded:

By focusing on this couple's immediate concerns and offering suggestions consistent with the clients' own ideas about change, they left with increased optimism and hope. They chose, at that time, not to schedule a return session. [...] In summary, walk-in services enhance accessibility of mental health counselling, take advantage of immediate client motivation, and are exceptionally cost efficient.

Numerous other walk-in SST cases are presented in Miller and Slive (2004), Bobele, Lòpez, Scamardo, and Solórzano (2008), Slive and Bobele (2011, 2018, in press b), Bobele and Slive (2014); and in a chapter by Bobele and several of his counseling students (Bobele et al., 2018) – also see Chapter 3 discussion of walk-in access.

Reflection question: How would service delivery (and social justice) be enhanced by removing barriers to therapy?

_____

_____

_____

_____

_____

_____

- Nancy McElheran (2021, in press; also see Clements, McElheran, Hackney, & Park, 2011) was one of the originators of the walk-in SST program at the Eastside Family Centre (EFC; now called the Eastside Community Mental Health Service) in Calgary, Canada, which has well-documented success. As she wrote (2021, p. 131):

> An outcome study conducted in 2015 indicated that the EFC serves the acute needs of an ethnically diverse population and that the therapy received significantly reduces distress, addresses the most pressing client concern(s), and offers useful ideas for clients to take away.

While the Eastside Centre has quantitatively and qualitatively reported many instructive instances of aiding clients to resolve problems in a single walk-in session, McElheran also notes (2021, p. 128) that:

> When identified, risk and safety issues are addressed directly by the therapist and team with a solution to the risk issue(s) emerging from the session. The solution could include the involvement of family members and/or Emergency Medical Services (EMS) assisting a client with getting to a hospital if that is required.

An example is provided by Janet Stewart et al. (2018) in which a walk-in client ("Tran") reported increasing imminent and alarming thoughts about killing his work supervisor. As they write (Stewart et al., 2018, pp. 85–86):

> During the intersession, the entire team was present for the discussion. [...] The decision to call the police was made collectively by the team. [...] The police supported the therapist and shift coordinator's decision to have Tran assessed at one of the local hospitals and stood by. [...] The therapist explained to Tran that the team could see how difficult his situation was and that we believed him when he told us that he was afraid he could act on his thinking. The therapist then explained that we were committed to keeping everyone safe, and that we would get Tran the help he was asking for. The therapist told Tran that the hospital would be able to help him. At that point, Tran began to cry and thanked us.

Reflection question: In addition to helping many clients to resolve problems in one session, how might a walk-in SST/OAAT service provide efficacious open access for other clients who may require more intensive and/or extensive assistance?

_____

_____

_____

_____

_____

_____

_____

_____

_____

- Jill Gibbons and Debbie Plath (2012) describe examples of using single session thinking in the context of their hospital medical work. They outline various practice guidelines:

  - Manage the immediate situation
  - Explain the system
  - Make an expert assessment
  - Set clear parameters and realistic goals for the session
  - Advocate for the client and negotiate with the system
  - Provide access to practical assistance
  - Provide information that can be accessed in the future
  - Review goals and resources as part of closure.

Reflection question: What one-session psychosocial intervention(s) might be useful for a patient in a hospital medical setting?

_____

_____

_____

_____

• Karen Story (2018) reports a case in which one family with a disabled parent (acquired brain injury) was seen for a total of 32 SSTs! After each session, when they were asked if they wanted to make another appointment, they responded: "Not now. This is what we need for now. We'll call when we're ready for another meeting." These repeated single sessions came to be called "coming in for tune-ups." Although OAAT, the family was seen, with varying combinations of attendees, over a five-year period an average of 6.5 times per year. Each session addressed different problems as determined by individual and family needs.

Recurrent SSTs are sometimes called *episodic, intermittent, repeat, booster, targeted,* or *catalytic* (see Budman, 1990; Cummings & Sayama, 1995; Hoyt, 1990/2017, 2000). Dryden (2023, in press) has proffered the term *ONEplus Therapy* – the *ONE* being the single planned session and the *plus* referring to the possibility of future conversations. Battino (2014, p. 405) refers to *sequential single session therapy* and Bobele et al. (2018, p. 234) refer to *serial single session therapy – SSST* either way! SST/OAAT does not necessarily mean "only one time"; as Jeff Young (2018) reports, perhaps 50% of "SST" clients eventually return for another session (or sessions), each of which can be approached as a complete stand-alone meeting. SST/OAAT is often useful when working with patients and families coping with new or ongoing medical-psychiatric problems. For example, for single session approaches with infants, see Birkin (2021); for the use of SST with families coping with a child's diagnosis of autism, see Rabba (2021); for SST with eating disorders, see Fleming (2021) and Barbara-May (2021); and for SST with people with a new HIV/AIDs diagnosis, see O'Loughin (2021). Rosenberg and McDaniel (2014) also discuss various ways clinicians can provide single session medical family therapy.

SSTs can thus be a useful part of a "family practitioner" model that replaces the notion of a definitive once-and-for-all "cure" with the more realistic and practical idea that patients/clients can return as needed throughout the life cycle. As I saw when working for many years at a staff-model health maintenance organization (Hoyt, 1995a, p. 30), in an intermittent model of therapy, the therapist will recede into the background until needed again; there is "interrupted continuity" (Morrill, 1978), the patient potentially having a series of brief treatment episodes over long periods (Anderson, 1981). The therapist-patient relationship may thus actually be long-term although frequently abeyant, with previous successful SST/brief therapy episodes setting a template for additional efficient work if/when the client returns. Arrangements to meet again with a particular clinician may be more easily made by appointment, assuming the clinician remains available long-term in the same delivery system; although walk-in SST arrangements may foster quicker access to care and if the same clinician is not on duty, a different practitioner can be informed about previous work by the client and by chart notes (see Chapter 3, "Access Options: SST/OAAT By Appointment or By Walk-In," pp. ___-___).

Reflection question: How can you both plan for a single session and let a client know that the door is open and that they can return on an as-needed basis?

_____

_____

_____

_____

_____

_____

- Victor Frankl (1963, pp. 178–179), in his classic book *Man's Search for Meaning: An Introduction to Logotherapy* describes a case in which in a single session he helped a man transform the meaning of suffering:

> Once, an elderly general practitioner consulted me because of his severe depression. He could not overcome the loss of his wife who had died two years before and whom he had loved above all else. Now how could I help him? What should I tell him? Well, I refrained from telling him anything, but instead confronted him with a question: 'What would have happened, Doctor, if you had died first, and your wife would have had to survive you?' 'Oh,' he said, 'for her this would have been terrible; how she would have suffered!' Whereupon I replied, 'You see, Doctor, such a suffering has been spared her, and it is you who have spared her this suffering: but now, you have to pay for it by surviving and mourning her.' He said no word but shook my hand and calmly left my office. Suffering ceases to be suffering in some way at the moment it finds a meaning, such as the meaning of a sacrifice.[3]

---

3   I am reminded of the lines in *Othello* (Act III, Scene 3, lines 92–93):

But I do love thee! and when I love thee not,
Chaos is come again.

> *Reflection question: What values does your client have that could be invoked in a single session to help them to see things in a different, meaningful, and more beneficial way?*
>
> _____
> _____
> _____
> _____
> _____
> _____

- Windy Dryden (2017) is his book *Single-Session Integrated CBT (SSI-CBT)* provides an excellent introduction to the use of Rational Emotive Behavior Therapy (REBT), a form of CBT, in SST. Indeed, in my back-cover endorsement of the book I wrote:

> Drawing from the work of Albert Ellis and others, this is *the* definitive guide to one-session work with clients using an active-directive problem-focused CBT approach. It also contains lots of ideas and practical tips that should be of interest for therapists of other theoretical persuasions wanting to help clients rapidly.

As Dryden (2017, p. 167; also see Dryden, 2020; Ellis & Dryden, 1987) notes:

> Epictetus's famous dictum, 'People are disturbed not by things, but by the views they take of them,' has been put forward as a saying that describes in a nutshell the role of cognition in the emotional disorders. In the ABC framework that most CBT therapists use, 'B' describes the cognitions that we hold about the adversity at 'A' that explain our responses to that adversity at 'C.'

> CBT is very well suited for use in SST and brief therapy (see Bond & Dryden, 2002). It is goal focused, systematic, and has specific methods. As Barnes, Carruthers, and Gigovic (2018, p. 178) noted, it is especially applicable if it can be determined that cognitive-behavioral issues "might be underpinning the individual's presenting concern. The most challenging aspect of the session involves finding the right fit between the interventions, the client's goal, and his/her readiness to engage in the suggested intervention."

Dryden (2020, p. 285) writes:

Developing a therapeutic alliance and helping clients become aware
that they have a choice in how to construe their reality and in their subsequent feelings and behaviors is empowering and opens the door for
better utilization of clients' resourcefulness (Hoyt & Berg, 1998/2000,
p.164). As contended by one of Dryden's main influences, Albert Ellis
(1998), REBT belongs in the constructivist camp in that it helps clients
to construct/build (not just uncover) a more functional sense of reality.

Dryden (2017) presents in detail the case of "Eugene," illustrating his
SSI-CBT process step-by-step:

✓   The first contact
✓   The pre-session phone call
✓   The face-to-face session – beginning, creating a focus, understanding
    the target problem, setting a goal, identifying the central mechanism,
    dealing with the central mechanism, making an impact, encouraging
    the client to apply learning inside and outside the session, summarizing,
    tidying up loose ends and the client's commitment to the future
✓   After the face-to-face session – reflection, providing a recording and
    transcript
✓   The follow-up session and evaluation.

Other case reports (e.g., Dryden, 2016, 2020, 2021; Ellis & Joffe, 2002)
also describe specific aspects of single session-REBT theory and practice.
For other CBT-based SST interventions, also see Öst et al. (2001; Ollendick & Davis, 2013), Robinson and Reiter (2016), Sperry and Binensztok
(2019), and Burns (2020).

Dryden (2021c) has also produced a book, *Help Yourself with Single-Session
Therapy*, in which he guides readers to apply single session principles to their
own problem solving.[4] Throughout the book, Dryden provides examples
and worksheets to help readers conceptualize and specify what they want to
achieve. Promoting application, he notes (p. 9) the difference "between reading this book and using it and will stress that only the latter will help you to
effect change." This is good advice for self-help readers and for therapists and

---

4   Talmon's (1993) *Single Session Solutions* is also intended as a self-help book based on SST principles. Preston, Varzos, and Liebert's (1995) *Every Session Counts: Making the Most of Your Brief
Therapy* also helps clients prepare for SST. Schleider's (2024) *Little Treatments, Big Effects: How to
Build Meaningful Moments that Can Transform Your Mental Health* describes various processes that
people can access on the internet and work through on their own.

their clients, regardless of particular theoretical orientation. I remember my grandmother admonishing me (drawing from her collection of Old World wisdom sayings), "If wishes were horses, beggars would ride."

Reflection questions: What would be some indications that SST CBT would be useful with a particular client? How might you proceed?

_____

_____

_____

_____

_____

_____

_____

- Flavio Cannistrà and Federico Piccirilli in their excellent book *Single-Session Therapy: Principles and Practice* (2018/2021a, p. 17) write: "SST's main strength lies in identifying and using the patient's resources and in blocking/modifying dysfunctional behaviors." The idea that the attempted unsuccessful solution actually perpetuates the problem is the basic concept from the Mental Research Institute (MRI) (see Watzlawick et al., 1974; Weakland & Fisch, 1992; Nardone & Salvini, 2018; Vitry, de Scorraille, & Hoyt, 2021a; Vitry, Scorraille, Portelli, & Hoyt, 2021b). Avoiding, stonewalling, insulting, accepting abuse, getting drunk, etc. don't usually solve problems. So, the therapist discerns what the client is doing that is *not* working and endeavors to get them to stop, because then they'll be more likely to do something new. (de Shazer's SFBT rule, "If it doesn't work don't do it again; do something else" is akin.) The basic MRI theory or mindset is to listen for, interdict, and block unsuccessful solutions attempts in order to get the person/couple/family to *stop not solving* the problem. As MRI therapists Richard Fisch and Karin Schlanger (1999, p. 2) wrote,

> Thus the thrust of therapy is not to get the complainants to do something so much as to stop what they have been doing about the problem. [...] In that sense, we would say that we don't treat problems, we treat attempted solutions.

As Cannistrà and Piccirilli (2018/2021, pp. 111–113) demonstrate, sometimes this can be accomplished in a single session. They describe seven key SST interventions:

1. Define the problem in practical terms – focusing the session so that the client sees and feels by the end of the session that they have worked on something specific that really matters to them.
2. Define the goal and identify priorities – what they will focus on in the meeting.
3. Ask for constant feedback – checking progress to ensure you are still on track to meet the goal helps maintain the alliance and maximizes the session's usefulness.
4. Investigate resources and exceptions to the problem – using what they already have as a starting point.
5. Investigate dysfunctional behavior – identify what does not help solve the problem.
6. Give feedback – with the primary aim of helping the client to notice present and past skills (as well as limitations).
7. Explain the open door – emphasize that while the endeavor is for single session, the client can return for a new appointment at any time.

In the same book, Veronica Torricelli (2018/2021, pp. 121–165) curates a collection of successful SST cases from the Italian Center for Single Session Therapy, including ones involving intrusive thoughts interfering with studying, improving romantic partner choices, a couple deciding to end their relationship, anger and detaching from an overly demanding father, stopping smoking and losing weight, sleep problems, sibling conflicts, use of SST in clinical supervision, reducing anxiety, family conflicts within the context of cancer treatment, helping someone to decide to "come out" to resolve their sexual identity, overcoming insecurity in the workplace, making career choices, setting a "final session" SST when ongoing progress is not being made, and adjusting to changing self-image. A wide range of techniques are skillfully used, including introducing the single session, defining the problem, clarifying the session goal and identifying priorities, exploring exceptions, considering dysfunctional behaviors, considering the client's theory of change, investigating internal and external resources, giving feedback, providing compliments, experimenting with new solutions in the session, and discussing next steps and the open door for possible return. As Torricelli writes in her concluding remarks (p. 165): "we believe that the cases show the range of possibilities SST offers, and the success that professionals can have in a single meeting."

Reflection question: By offering (but not insisting on) the possibility of an SST, a wide range of clients have been helped to achieve their immediate goals – and some of the clients have later gone on to pursue more therapy. What are some cases that you have had that resulted in perhaps an unexpected success in a single session?

_____

_____

_____

_____

_____

_____

_____

_____

_____

_____

- Giorgio Nardone and Claudette Portelli (2005, p. 50) report that:

> During these last 15 years, at CTS [Centro di Terapia Strategica, in Arezzo, Italy] we have treated thousands of patients with phobic and obsessive disorders. [...] At present, the efficacy of the advanced treatment model for anxiety, phobia, and panic attacks [is] in 50 percent of these cases there were no traces of relevant symptoms after the first session.

Nardone and his group draw upon earlier work that Nardone did with Paul Watzlawick (Nardone & Watzlawick, 1990, 2005). In an interview with Watzlawick (Hoyt, 1998a/2001, p. 147), Paul remarked:

> In my view, the most frequent factor that brings about change in human lives is what Franz Alexander called a *corrective emotional experience* [...] 'Insight' may very well (and often does) *follow* change – which makes it into a consequence and not a cause.

Paul went on (in Hoyt, 1998a/2001, p. 149) to say:

> One of the basic principles of systems theory is that every system is its *own best* explanation [...] What matters to me (exclusively) is the patient's specific problem; and what he has done so far to 'solve it,' i.e., the *attempted solution*, which in our perspective is the main factor that maintains and exacerbates the problem.

and (on p. 151):

> As far as constructivism is concerned, only the *name* is modern. That our views of reality are *subjective* and by no means an objective 'true' view has been postulated by philosophers (e.g., Vico, Kant, Schopenhauer, Jaspers), by physicists (e.g., Einstein, Heisenberg, Schrodinger), and even mathematicians. [...] Constructivism [...] makes a clear distinction between reality of the *first order* (as conveyed to us by our sensory organs in terms of perceptions) and reality of the *second order* (i.e., the meaning, significance, and value that every one of us inevitably attributes to the first-order reality – which remains totally subjective, unprovable, and, therefore, the cause of human conflict and misunderstandings).[5]

Applying these constructivist concepts, Nardone and Portelli (2005) describe the basis of their advanced strategic therapy model (p. 4):

> A strategic psychotherapist is not interested in discovering deep realities and the *why* of things, but only *how* things work and how to make them work as well as possible. Our first concern is to adapt our knowledge to the partial 'realities' that we need to work on, developing strategies based on the objectives to be reached, that can be adapted step by step to the evolutions of 'reality.'

and (on p. 5):

> We therefore avoid [...]. trying to determine a definitive, universal mode of intervention. It is always the solution that adapts to the problem and not the contrary [...] In short, strategic logic wants to be flexible and tries to adapt to its object of study.

Toward this goal, they have developed a "strategic dialogue" (pp. 36–37; also see Nardone & Salvini, 2018). Nardone and Portelli detail a case (2005, pp. 39–46) in which an obsessive-phobic patient's "fear of losing control *makes* him lose control, until he is overwhelmed by panic." They note (2005, p. 42):

> So, through these change-oriented questions, the person will come to feel that what he previously thought of as being helpful [avoidance],

---

5   Thus, Shakespeare said: "There is nothing either good or bad, but thinking makes it so" (*Hamlet*, Act II, Scene 2); and de Shazer (1993) wrote "Creative misunderstanding: There is no escape from language." For more on constructivism and therapy, see Watzlawick (1978, 1984), Watzlawick, Beavin, and Jackson (1967), Watzlawick et al. (1972); and Hoyt (1994c, 1996c, 1998b).

in reality is rendering him always more frustrated since this confirms his incapacity to overcome his fear.

and, on p. 43:

> In therapy, it is important that the patient should *feel* that something has to change, rather than merely understand it. [...] What triggers off the change process is our feeling, our perception; all the rest will then follow. One can well understand that one needs to change, but one needs to feel it in order to start doing something about it. Once this emotional recognition is accomplished, the therapist can proceed in being more 'directive' and thus give prescriptions. The patient will be more willing to accept and follow them.

In another case, reported at the 4th International SST Symposium in Rome, Nardone (in press) described a single session with a young man who had developed the belief that his father wanted to poison him. In one family meeting, Nardone gets the father to agree to serve as a taster of the son's food, an act that not only logically demonstrates that the food is not poisoned but also has significant emotional impact because it undeniably shows the father's love (not enmity). The son abandons the filicide delusion.

Reflection question: How can you appeal to a reluctant SST client's emotions in a way that will facilitate their engaging in difficult new behaviors?

- Martin Söderquist (2023, p. 22) describes the approach taken by him and his Couple Counselling Team in Malmö, Sweden:

> In my colleagues and my version of [SST/OAAT] with couples are thinking and practice [which] include a preference for therapist as

non-expert, focusing doing and present-future most of the time. Sometimes couples present problems that need more attention than just being mentioned and the couples are in the front seat – we are to follow their lead. The focus of the OAAT session will still be on present situation and hopes for the session. SST/OAAT is very different from many couple therapy models which often are grounded in theories, problem focused and built on several sessions. The thinking and practice of OAAT with couples [... includes] no serial thinking and focusing the session today.

As Söderquist et al. (2021, p. 165, italics in original) wrote earlier:

Although brief relational work is now accepted, going from *brief* to *OAAT* relational work, beginning in the 1990–2000s, was another giant leap. Going from serial thinking about processes to *one-off sessions in OAAT* is a great challenge. The idea of scheduling one session, collaboratively doing the best in that session and leaving the decision to the client – to make a new appointment, to find another counselor, or to take care of their situation on their own – is for many couple therapists very much 'outside the box.'

A good theory is a map that leads us somewhere useful (Hoyt, 2017, p. 186). Leonardo da Vinci (1452–1519; quoted in Nardone & Portelli, 2005, p. 1) said "Good practice does not exist without good theory." Kurt Lewin (Marrow, 1977) averred, "There is nothing as practical as a good theory." The Malmö group has a broad background of training (including strategic family therapy, family play therapy, emotionally focused therapy, the Gottman Method). Söderquist (2023, p. 53) writes:

We all have found that the solution-focused model is highly suitable when doing OAAT sessions, and we integrate our OAAT mindset with our special trainings and interests. Our guiding principles in OAAT:

✓ Having a choice
✓ Couples have different reasons for scheduling a session
✓ Couples know how best to move forward after the session
✓ Couples have hopes and goals for the OAAT session
✓ Context marking is of utmost importance
✓ Start from scratch knowing nothing about the couple in advance
✓ Being able to be genuinely surprised and giving hope.

Söderquist (2018, 2023; Söderquist et al., 2021) present a series of SST/OAAT cases to illustrate their work with couples presenting a variety of issues.

Reflection questions: How does the theoretical frame(s) you use help you to do successful SSTs? What assumptions/mindsets are included in your preferred frame(s)?

_____

_____

_____

_____

_____

_____

_____

_____

- Karen Young (2018; also see 2011a, 2011b, 2017; Duvall, Young, & Kays-Burden, 2012) describes the growth of narrative therapy walk-in clinics in Ontario, Canada. Narrative therapy was first developed by Michael White and David Epston (1990; White, 2007; also see Freedman & Combs, 1996; Hoyt, 2001d; Duvall & Beres, 2011; Denborough, 2014; Madigan, 2019; Cooper, 2024, in press). Describing the narrative therapy theoretical orientation and its SST utility, Karen Young writes (2018, p. 62):

> It is a collaborative, non-pathologizing and competency-focused approach to therapy. It is based on the notion that stories are created to make sense of our lives, and that the stories we create then also influence our lives and relationships. Problems are viewed as separate from people's identities and part of the larger context of people's lives. People are seen as having knowledge, skills, abilities, values, and commitments that can assist them to respond to the problems that are influencing their lives.

She provides (2018, pp. 64–66) a 9-step guideline structure for walk-in sessions influenced by brief narrative therapy:

(1) Pre-session preparation: looking carefully at the client's pre-session questionnaire for preferences, hopes, and values; ideas about possible externalizing language for the problem; and glimmers of stories, knowledge, and skills.

(2) Beginning the session: the counselor explaining processes, procedures, and purposes.

(3) Setting the agenda: "I am prepared to work hard with you for the next hour or so in relation to what it is that brought you here. What should we focus on in our conversation so that you leave feeling it was useful?"

(4) Discovering strengths: Consistent with the narrative therapy principle that *the person is not the problem,* seeking permission from the client to pause problem talk and explore strengths, skills, abilities, knowledge, preferences, etc.

(5) Exploring the problem: Asking questions to both understand the client's understanding of the problem and to create different, novel ways of viewing the problem.

(6) Developing details of knowledge, skills, values, and preferences: Thickening the path, how and why they want to move toward preferences and any ways they already are doing so.

(7) Reviewing and expanding what was useful: collaboratively exploring what has been helpful in the conversation.

(8) Co-developing next steps: Discussing how to keep the ideas/plans going and what supports may be helpful.

(9) Wrapping up: The counselor provides a summary report and any documents collaboratively developed (e.g., see Cooper & "Ariane," 2018; Cooper, in press), offers to tell clients what effects they have had on the counselor (what will be remembered and has been learned from them), and the client is asked to privately complete session evaluation.

Scot Cooper (2024, in press) also provides an extensive account of how narrative therapy principles can inform SST practice. He notes (2024, p. 18) that "brevity comes about as a consequence of how we think about people, problems, change, and therapy and how these premises shape what we do." Employing a mindset that strongly favors clients' local knowledge and preferred ways of seeing themselves (rather than a pathologizing discourse), he highlights and illustrates concepts such as meaning-making, storying, curiosity (wonder and exploration), use of questions, languaging, generating local knowledge, problems as outside of people (externalization), identity projects, therapist position/being in the conversation, use of take-home documents, rites of passage (separation phase, transitional/liminal phase, reincorporation phase), and therapy as a definitional ceremony.

Reflection questions: Since "the stories we tell ourselves and each other do much to influence what we see and what we do" (Hoyt, 2017, p. 230) and "some stories are better than others" (Hoyt, 2000a), how can narrative practices be used as an "archeology of hope" (Monk, Winslade, Crocket, & Epston, 1996) to bring forth strengths, preferences, and energy to help people get more of what they want? How might you use narrative concepts with a particular SST client?

_____

_____

_____

_____

_____

_____

_____

_____

- The Redecision Therapy model of Mary Goulding and Robert Goulding (1979; also see Hoyt, 1995d/2001; 2017, pp. 51–53; and Hoyt & Cannistrà, 2023a, pp. 92–100) draws on transactional analysis (TA) theory and Gestalt techniques, as well as the Gouldings' own innovations, to rapidly generate powerful and potentially life-changing therapeutic experiences. The Redecision Therapy model involves a thinking structure with a number of key elements: contact; contract; con; chief bad feelings, thoughts, behaviors, and psychosomatics; chronic games, belief systems, and fantasies; childhood early decisions; impasse resolution; and maintaining the victory. Their key contract question, _What are you willing to change today?_ contains all the elements of brief and single session therapy in one pithy sentence!

What = specificity, target, focus

are = active verb, present tense

you = self as agent, personal functioning

willing = choice, responsibility, initiative

to change = alter or be different, not just "work on" or "explore"

today = now, in the moment

_?_ = inquiry, open field, therapist inviting and receptive but not insistent.

Goulding and Goulding (1979, pp. 280–281) wrote:

Redecision is a beginning rather than an ending. After redecision the person begins to think, feel, and behave in new ways. At this point he may decide to terminate therapy. We applaud this choice. Our philosophy of treatment is that therapy should be as condensed and quick as possible and that termination is a triumph, like graduation.

Mary Goulding (1990, pp. 307–308) elaborated:

To help the client effect personal changes in the shortest possible time, the therapist must work precisely and efficiently, focusing only on material that is relevant to the contract. […] I am impressed with the fact that clients continue to make important changes after therapy has ended, if they have learned to believe in their own ability to change their lives.

In the case of "Anne" presented in the professional training videotape *Redecision Therapy* (Goulding & Goulding, 1988), we see them work in a single session with a woman troubled by feelings of incompetency. Rather than working within a psychodynamic transference model, in which the therapist becomes the participant-observer "object," or within a cognitive-behavioral model, in which the therapist becomes an instructor or editor of the client's thoughts, here the client is encouraged to do two-chair Gestalt work. In the second chair, she undergoes a "Parent Interview" (McNeel, 1976) in which she "becomes" her father (extrojecting the introject, so to speak) and then engages in a powerful dialogue with him in which she experiences and realizes the futility of trying to remain an incompetent child to please her father. Her therapeutic impasse is resolved as she externalizes and disengages from her sense of incompetency. Back in her Adult self after the exercise, she processes the experience to gain further insight and a sense of autonomy and self-mastery.

Reflection question: What role-play or enactment could vivify for one (or more) of your SST clients how they are "stuck" and what they need to do to get "unstuck"?

_____

_____

_____

_____

_____

_____

_____

- Solution Focused Brief Therapy (SFBT; also called Solution Focused Therapy, SFT) was originated by Steve de Shazer, Insoo Kim Berg, and others (see de Shazer, 1988, 1991; Berg & Miller, 1992; de Shazer et al., 2007) at the Brief Family Therapy Center in Milwaukee, Wisconsin. It is a non-normative, constructivist view that emphasizes the use of language in the social construction of reality. Operating from the assumption that clients have competencies, it uses questions to help clients shift perspectives to focus on resources – a very useful approach when attempting to assist clients in a single session. The three "basic rules" of SFBT (de Shazer, quoted in Hoyt, 1996, p. 68; see de Shazer et al., 2007, pp. 1–3):

(1) If it ain't broke, don't fix it
(2) Once you know what works, do more of it, and
(3) If it doesn't work, don't do it again; do something different.

Seven basic questions were developed to organize the SFBT conversation, which is intended to highlight descriptions of (and bring about) clients' "best hopes" and desired outcomes:

✓ *Miracle Question:*_"Suppose that one night, while you were asleep, there was a miracle and this problem was solved. How would you know? What would be different?"

✓ *Formula First-Session Task*: "Between now and next time we meet, I would you like you to observe, so that you can describe to me next time, what happens in your [*pick one*: family, life, marriage, relationship] that you want to continue to have happen."

✓ *Goal-Building Questions*: "What brings you here today? How can I be helpful to you? What changes have you noticed since you first made the call to set up this appointment? What needs to happen here so that when you leave you will think, 'It was good that we went to see the therapist?' What will tell you that you're on track?"

✓ *Exceptions Questions*: "When in the past might the problem have happened, but didn't? What is different about those times when the problem does not happen?"

✓ *Efficacy (Agency) Questions*: "How did you do that? How did you get that to happen? What was each of you doing differently when you were doing better?"

✓ *Endurance (Coping) Questions*: "Given the terrible situation, how come things aren't worse? How have you managed to cope as well as you have?"

✓ *Scaling Questions*

Hope: On a scale from 1 to 10, 1 being absolutely no hope and 10 being complete confidence, what number would you give your current level of hope? What will tell you that your level has gone up one level? What number will be high enough to warrant your working hard to try and change things?

Motivation: On a scale from 1 to 10, 1 being no motivation and completely ready to give up and 10 being willing to do anything to achieve your goals, what number would you give your current level of motivation?

Progress: On a scale from 1 to 10, where 1 is the problem at its worse and 10 is the day after the miracle, what number would you give your current level of progress? What number will tell you that you have made enough progress so that you can consider it solved?

Insoo Berg and Yvonne Dolan (2001, p. 1) wrote:

If we had to define the SFBT approach in one sentence without talking about philosophy or techniques, we would describe it as 'the pragmatics of hope and respect.' Rather than focusing on deficits, SFBT therapists view clients as competent and in possession of resources. SFBT therapists do not attempt to educate or 'enlighten' clients; instead, they prefer to view clients as having positive rather than negative intentions. Completely accepting of the client's view, the SFBT therapist uses the client's perceptions as valuable resources to help create the change the client desires.

Discussing the SFBT "nonexpert stance," de Shazer et al. (2007, p. 155) advised:

In debating the issue of what differentiates SFBT from other approaches, one seasoned solution-focused therapist suggested that one would not see a solution-focused therapist give advice. This brought a quizzical look to Insoo's face. 'What?' she said. 'You mean that if you knew something that would help the client, you wouldn't tell them?' The solution-focused conviction that clients have the information they need to design and achieve the desired outcome can sometimes be taken to mean that the therapist never offers ideas, suggestions, or alternatives during a therapeutic conversation. This isn't necessarily the case. However, there are two caveats about advice-giving from a SFBT perspective. [...] First, compared to skill-training or deficit-remediating approaches, advice-giving doesn't happen often in SFBT. The client is the first and foremost authority on where they want to go and how to get there. [...] Second, the SFBT therapist's suggestions are simply that – suggestions. They are offered tentatively, as alternatives the client may adopt or discard depending on whether or not they fit. [And, continuing on p. 156] Our job is not to think up the right solutions for our clients and to convince them to accept them. Our job is to create the conditions under which clients find their own solutions, to help clients look into their hearts to find what they truly want and how they might get there.

And he (de Shazer et al., 2007, p. 160) clarified:

Any technique that requires a directive or expert stance on the part of the therapist or that compromises the client's ability to choose the direction of the therapy is not compatible with SFBT and should not be used if one wishes to maintain a solution-focused stance.

SFBT has a broad, international following. BRIEF (formerly called the Brief Therapy Practice), based in London (England), is the premier group offering SFBT (George, Iveson, & Ratner, 1990; Ratner, George, & Iveson, 2012; Ratner & Yusef, 2015). They have been raising questions about what is truly essential to SFBT. Shennan and Iveson (2012, p. 294) describe their group's research-supported evolution that has resulted in the gradual elimination of various practices that were previously thought to be essential but were found not to be. These include: (1) dropping the categorization of client-therapist relationships as either *customer, complainant,* or *visitor* and instead assuming that the client is motivated and that it is the therapist's job to help the client find what he or she is motivated for; (2) working toward the client's "hopes" rather than "problem resolution"; (3) inviting detailed descriptions of "preferred futures" rather than setting "goals"; (4) focusing on "instances where the preferred future is happening" rather than on "descriptions of the problem"; (5) elimination of the in-session planning break; (6) dropping end-of-session tasks and focusing more on in-session conversations; and (7) providing summaries rather than compliments. Connie and Froerer (2023) describe further developments that emphasize the use of language co-construction to highlight client agency and desired outcomes. This is part of the movement toward "SFBT 2.0" (McKergow, 2016, 2021).

The focus of SFBT remains on solutions – on *what works for clients.* For more about SFBT/SFT, see de Shazer and Berg references plus Ziegler and Hiller (2001), Bannink (2011), Ratner et al. (2012), Hoyt (2015),

McKergow (2021), Connie and Froerer (2023), and Murphy (2024). As Murphy (2024, p. 8) writes:

> SFT is brief by design versus default, and every session is approached as if it were the last. This practical mindset expedites change by keeping therapists and clients on track. It also explains why SFT techniques are commonly used in single-session therapy (Hoyt et al., 2018).

Chris Iveson, Evan George, and Harvey Ratner (2014) present an example of a single-session solution-focused therapy with a troubled young woman done as a demonstration at a workshop. The session starts (p. 331) with the therapist asking, "What are your best hopes from this meeting?" and when she replies that she was "intrigued," the therapist follows with "And if being intrigued turns out to be a good idea what do you hope it might lead to?" and she replies, "A better future for my kids; a better future for me." As the session continues, the therapist asks (p. 332): "So let's imagine a little miracle happens tonight and it stops the past messing with your future so you are no longer being held back from where you want to be – " and the client interjects with the beginning of a sense of wonderment: "—I don't know what I'd do with it" and the therapist persists: "What's the first thing you'd notice when you woke up tomorrow that somehow gave you the first hint that the past was no longer messing with your future?" In their commentary (p. 335), Iveson et al. note:

> Her response is marked by an almost palatable sense of excitement on her part, a sense of wonder, that we can imagine is very different from the client's response were she to be asked to describe what is bothering her. (Hoyt, 2009a, p. 184, describes this as enhancing *'solution sight.'*) The sort of description that the therapist appears to be prioritizing through his questioning is rooted in the client's everyday reality; it may be a miracle that she is considering, but this is a miracle that is happening within her daily routine, within her home, with her children present as witnesses and participants.

Later (p. 337) they comment: "The therapist is persistent, inviting the client into describing multiple layers of difference" and (p. 341)

> perhaps what is particularly striking is the therapist's refusal to blur the picturing by suggesting at any time that the client should take action, should put into practice any of these different ways of living.

He sticks purely at deriving description and nothing else. There is no pressure, no problem-solving, no action-oriented suggestions.

They report (p. 344) that a six-month follow-up from the referring social worker indicated

> Over the next few weeks after having the session with you I saw a dramatic change in her confidence and ability to prioritize and effectively deal with situations. I saw her planning for a future she used to dread […] she was thinking forwards, planning for her children's needs and was emotionally far more resilient and calm.

In another single-session SFBT case, Iveson (2019) saw a suicidal 19-year-old woman in hospital for one session which was focused on helping her move from a despairing "I don't do hope" to descriptions of (p. 132) "So, let's imagine that you wake up tomorrow feeling less pain, less stress – what would you notice instead?" The single session was a significant positive turning point for the woman – eight years later, she was married and had two children. In concluding, Iveson (p. 132) notes:

> It can be argued that Solution-Focused Brief Therapy has only three questions:

✓ What are your best hopes from our work together?
✓ How will your life be different if these hopes are realized?
✓ What are you already doing or have done in the past that might help bring these hopes to fruition?

Reflection question: What are some questions you might ask to help an SST client to focus on his/her/their hopes, what he/she/they may already be doing in that direction, and ways to achieve them?

_____
_____
_____
_____
_____
_____
_____

- Franz Alexander (Alexander & French, 1946; discussed in Hoyt, Rosenbaum, & Talmon, 1992, p. 83), describing the concept of the *corrective emotional experience*, cited the classic example from Victor Hugo's novel, *Les Misérables*, of the convicted thief, Jean Valjean, who stole from the bishop who befriended him. As may be recalled, when the bishop forgave him, Valjean had a conversion experience, apparently transforming from sinner to saint. To understand this apparent "Single Session Therapy," we need to consider two items that Alexander does not mention. First, we should recognize why Valjean was in prison in the first place: for stealing bread to feed a hungry child. Second, later in the story, Valjean himself offers unexpected forgiveness to the sadistic Javert, who has been his jailor and persecutor. Rather than triggering another happy conversation, however, Javert commits suicide by throwing himself from a bridge. Why does one kind act succeed while the other doesn't? The story is fictional and such motivations are usually multidetermined, but an important key might be the existence of underlying cognitive schemata. SST and brief therapy are more likely to produce dramatic shifts if favorable latent mental images are already in place, waiting (ready) to be re-evoked (see Short, 2022). The bishop's kindness toward Valjean (a "good thief" who had stolen to feed a child) reminded Valjean of his own goodness, whereas kindness toward Javert only met a hard heart and evoked more shame and rage. The experience might be so "corrective" only if the recipient is open (ready) for healing.[6]

Reflection question: What is good in the client that can be (re)activated, perhaps in one session?

_____

_____

_____

_____

_____

_____

_____

---

6   The terms *heal, whole, health, hale,* and *holy* all derive from the same old Middle English and Anglo-Saxon words (*hole, hale*). (Hoyt, 2017, p. 133).

- Hillary Keeney and Brad Keeney (2019; also see 2014) recount a one-session demonstration interview (conducted at a workshop in Hungary) with a man with a skin condition, in which they creatively and humorously engage with him, suggesting different ideas and getting him to laughingly entertain the (reframed) possibility that his dermatological problem might actually be a kind of blessed stigmata on his way to sainthood. They write (2019, pp. 134–135):

> Our orientation [...] regards each session's structure as a three-act play that improvisationally unfolds from an entrenched beginning, to a transformational middle, and finally to an expanded ending where more possibilities and greater creative energy are found [...] what we sometimes simply refer to as going from a 'small room' to a big room. Clients come seeking change – movement from their current impoverished situation to one that is more resourceful, interesting, expansive, and full of life. [...] Rather than joining clients in perpetuating the same way of first knowing and then subsequently acting in relationship to their life circumstance, we immediately hunt for any opportunity to make an exit toward new territory without preconceived notions of how we will get there and what will arise along the way. Creative change lies outside the box of both the practitioner's and client's knowing, and that fertile ground is only reached by surrendering to the great mind and dance of interaction.

They also advise (2019, p. 142):

> Every session is an opportunity to uncover the mystery of the greater whole of life that remains hidden when held inside impoverished frames and shrunken contexts.

Reflection question: What is something unusual you could do to help an SST client shift to a different, more playful and salutary view of their situation?

_____

_____

_____

_____

_____

_____

_____

_____

- David Keith (2019) describes an SST by proxy. He advised a physician colleague what to say in one session to an 83-year-old widowed, very anxious woman who was trying to run a large family business and deal with her dead husband's possessions. She didn't have the appropriate skills but was resisting turning power over to her highly qualified sons. She would call her sons for advice – but then repeatedly dismiss their suggestions. To help the lady see the absurd untenability of her position, Keith advised his colleague to suggest to the lady (p. 147):

> This certainly is a difficult set of problems for you to be dealing with all by yourself. It sounds like you are stuck with being father, mother and CEO. And you are so isolated! I guess one solution would be to get a partner, a new husband maybe? One possibility is that I could marry you. But my wife wouldn't like that. I would have to divorce her first. I am not sure she would think much of the idea. Or, I could arrange for you to adopt me and make me the oldest son, but I know your sons would be upset if I tried to be their boss.

Three weeks later, Keith heard from his colleague, who had nervously said almost word-for-word to the woman what Keith had suggested. The colleague reported that the sons had called and had said that the woman was much better – much less anxious, fewer phone calls, easier to talk with. Drawing on his perspective (Keith, 2015) of symbolic and experiential family relational systems, in his conclusion he comments (p. 148):

> My view is that my clumsy absurd remark [including what Keith calls 'therapeutic teasing'] affected her symbolic (subjective) organization: it had an extra-intellectual effect in the realm of symbolic experience and provided what turned out to be a refreshing immersion in absurdity.

Reflection question: In his Pensées, *the French mathematician and philosopher Blaise Pascal (1632–1662) said, "The heart has its reasons which reason knows nothing of. [...] We know the truth not only by the reason, but by the heart." When might love and humor get you and an SST client to a good place beyond rationality?*

```
_____
_____
_____
_____
_____
```

- Jeffrey Kottler (2019) reports a one-session meeting "when impatience gets the best of me." He got so frustrated with a disingenuous client that he told the man that he couldn't be helped and that he would get worse. After the session, Kottler felt chagrined by his outburst – of all the excellent therapies Kottler had studied, he said (p. 160), "not a single one resulted from laziness, frustration, or impatience." Only years later did Kottler learn from someone that after the session the client, having been told that he was a hopeless case, was so upset that he went out to his car where he reached for a vial of cocaine in the glove compartment. Kottler's informant went on (p. 61):

> But then you scared the shit out of him so badly that he opened the window and threw the vial away. He told me from that moment he never touched the stuff again. Went cold turkey. Anyway, he wanted me to thank you for what you did.

Long ago, D.W. Winnicott (1949), in his classic paper "Hate in the Countertransference," described the value of the therapist's genuineness. I have come to sometimes think of countertransference as "client-inspired therapist contributions" (Hoyt, 2001c/2017).

Reflection question: Have you ever gotten so frustrated that you told the unvarnished truth and it was your authenticity that helped the client? What happened?

```
_____
_____
_____
_____
_____
_____
_____
_____
```

• When I was a predoctoral intern at the University of Wisconsin-Madison, I once followed Carl Whitaker to the E.R. (as reported in Hoyt, 2017, pp. 308–309) to watch him interview a teenage girl who had taken a little overdose to spite the boyfriend who had just dumped her. Carl asked her a series of questions, like if she were dead who would get her favorite hairbrush? Who would get her clothes? How long did she think it would take before the ex-boyfriend was dating someone else? etc. etc. She got self-righteously incensed and declared, "My sister's not going to get my favorite brush, and I'm not gonna let that goddamn #%&#%$# have the satisfaction of seeing me dead!" A few more minutes and we discharged her from the E.R. as "no longer a threat to self."

Elsewhere (Hoyt & Cannistrà, 2023, pp. 55–56), I have described a single session meeting with a young woman embarking on an eating disorder in which I portrayed to her the probable negative consequences so dramatically that she got "scared straight" and stopped the problematic behavior. One could also ask "The Nightmare Question" (Reuss, 1997): "Suppose tonight, while you're sleeping, the problem gets worse…"; or use the "How Worse Technique" (Fisch et al., 1982; Nardone & Watzlawick, 1990) that asks the client what actions he or she would need to do to make their problem worse. For some other examples of provocative SST interventions in potentially risky circumstances, along with discussions of appropriate cautions, see Bobele (1987, 1988; Weakland, 1988). Monte Bobele (1987 and reprised 2019, pp. 38–40), and I (Hoyt, 2017, p. 246) each independently, when we could not rationally persuade vengeful clients not to harm someone, instead got them to not assault the other persons by using their anger as a resource, convincing them that the other persons would suffer more if never attacked and thus have to live in perpetual uncertainty and fear. Milton Erickson (see Haley, 1973, pp. 270–273) and Frank Farrelly and Jeff Brandsma (1974) also reported successful SSTs using provocative methods.

Reflection questions: When might you use provocation with an SST client? What safeguards would be important to minimize the possibility that a challenging SST approach might make things worse (not better)?

_____

_____

_____

_____

_____

```
_____
_____
_____
_____
_____
```

- Eric Greenleaf (2013) gifted us beautiful descriptions of how three different people (one of them himself) dealt, each in their own way, successfully with serious illnesses. In one of the cases, "Judy" describes meeting with Eric for a single session after receiving a diagnosis of advanced breast cancer. She was distressed, and she was not particularly interested in cultivating a "positive attitude" (p. 103):

> They all want me to think 'positive.' They say it will cure me. Everyone's always telling me about some aunt of theirs, or someone, who cured herself of breast cancer by having a positive attitude. Supposedly, I'm doing this wrong. But damn it, it's not my fault that I have this, and it's not going to be my fault if I die from it. The way everyone thinks I'm supposed to do this, it's not my way. I'm not that kind of a person. I'm a pessimist. I'm a lawyer, a litigator. You get your case ready, you work it up as well as you can, but you have to know your odds of winning, or losing. You can't lose sight of the worst-case scenario – or the best-case either, for that matter. You have to settle if your case is shit.

Eric pointed out: "You don't get to settle here, do you?" and Judy replies "No, so I have to be ready for the worst. And I have no idea how to do that." To which Eric replied: "No one knows what will happen. And so you have to prepare for life. And you have to prepare for death." He then advised her on how to prepare for death: getting affairs in order, finishing projects, supporting and making memories for her children, sharing fears and worries and telling the children she loves them, doing whatever art she does, celebrating what needs celebrating, pruning unnecessary things and people. "You have to keep living while you're living." And then he tells her: "To prepare for life, you have to get your affairs in order. You have to complete projects. You have to make memories for your children…" and repeats the same list. Essentially, he appreciates and uses as a resource that she is tough-minded, that she said "You get your case ready, you work it up as well as you can […] You can't lose sight of the worst-case scenario – or the best case either, for that matter." Judy followed her path with heart. Nine years later, in good health and having sent her second daughter off to college, Judy wrote an unpublished memoir describing the SST with Eric.

Reflection question: How can the person's style and predilections be utilized to help them go where they want to go?

_____

_____

_____

_____

_____

_____

_____

_____

_____

- Rubin Battino (2014) has described examples of a variety of SST approaches, including Guided Imagery Therapy (GIT; Battino, 2000, 2020). Based on the Gouldings' (1979) basic contract question, *"What are you willing to change today?"* he notes regarding GIT (Battino, 2021, p. 42):

  I need just four bits of information:

  1. *A brief statement of what troubles the client.* (I consistently avoid the word "problem." My clients have things that *bother* or *trouble* or *concern* them.)
  2. *Relaxation* – Do they have a preferred method of relaxing or meditating, and what is it?
  3. *Safe haven* – Do they have special safe and secure place that they can go to within their mind that is real or imaginary?
  4. *Healing Entity* – What or who do they feel will help them through this troubled time and into their future?

  He goes on to write (2021, p. 42):

  Please note that the client supplies all of the information needed to realistically help them through their current difficulties. *They know* what changes are possible in their lives. There is no easy way for the therapist to know enough about the client to find ways of guiding them or making practical suggestions in the first (and maybe only) session that you are with them. So, in the GIT method *the client tells you* exactly what will help them! Your job, then, is to basically tell them all of this back, in a detailed and suggestive manner. That is, you *guide* them through their own change process. [...] The delivery of steps 2–4 are generally via hypnosis. (The delivery can also be made in other styles as in simply telling stories.)

Recently, Battino has begun to experiment with Multiple Issue Psychotherapy (MIP). He (2022) reports the case of "Anabel" (who in one session successfully addressed sadness over the end of a two-year relationship, PTSD, and headbanging and scratching). In another case report, Battino (2023, pp. 40–41) describes "Mike," who successfully resolved various stress, anxiety, and depression issues in one visit. Generally speaking, SST therapists are advised to collaborate with the client to prioritize goals and determine which problem is to be the specific focus of the session. There are reports, however, such as these by Battino and those described in Miller and C'de Baca (2001) in which epiphanies and sudden insights remove multiple problems in a single session.

Reflection question: How about a "two-fer"? How could you help a client to address and resolve more than one problem in the same single session?

- A somewhat related hypnotherapy method of "natural problem-solving" involves Ernest Rossi's (Rossi & Cheek, 1988; Rossi, 1996) Mirroring Hands Technique, which has been described and elaborated by Richard

Hill and Ernest Rossi (2017) in *The Practitioner's Guide to Mirroring Hands*.[7] They begin (pp. 1–3) by describing a "walk-in" experience with a woman who had arrived unexpectedly looking for help. Hill reports:

> She was very expressive with her hands, pushing them toward me to highlight things as she spoke. I was suddenly transported to my workshops with Ernest Rossi. This looked something like what happens during a Mirroring Hands experience. [...]
>
> *I've noticed that you are very expressive with your hands. Have you ever really looked at your hands ...noticed what is really interesting about them?*
>
> [...] As the experience unfolded, she told me, with some surprise, that she felt her hands were representing two aspects of her persona. One hand was representing a part of herself she keeps private and the other hand was representing her public face. It was like watching someone open doors to rooms she had not seen for a long time. Sometimes she shared what was happening and other times she just explored her 'rooms' privately. Many things happened over the next 30 minutes [...] but finally her hands settled together, with her 'public self' hand totally covering her 'private self' hand. [...] It was clear that she knew something now that she did not know 30 minutes ago [...] She had allowed her hands to become mirrors into her deeper self. [...] The most amazing thing is that she did the bulk of this work without my interference, imposition, or direction. She found what she was searching for: how to begin her own healing. I expect she might say that was 60 minutes that truly changed her life.

As Hill and Rossi (2017, p. 44) note and elaborate, the groundwork for this SST method involves three key elements:

---

7   I saw Richard Hill (2018) do a very skillful single-session demonstration of the "mirroring hands" method in which, rather than just guiding the client into a chair, Richard asked in which chair the person would feel more ready to make a change. Before, I would automatically ask/direct a client to sit in the chair that I had set across from me. I still have my customary office seat, but I learned that even how we sit down is important. One can create a different dynamic by asking the client to make themselves comfortable so that they feel ready to work on whatever problem has brought them to therapy. The difference may seem subtle, but the latter attends to the alliance by respectfully inviting and utilizing the client's responsiveness in a more relational and emergent way that helps to co-create the therapeutic experience.

It is important to recognize that therapy begins at first encounter – or even before, when the client begins to think about possibly seeing a therapist. As Marshall McLuhan (quoted in Karrass, 1992, p. 78) cautioned, for better or worse: "The spell can occur immediately upon contact, as in the first bars of a melody."

1. Focused attention
2. Curiosity – for information, playfulness, and meaning
3. Nascent confidence (confidence in the potential of the process).

There is much that could be said, and interested readers are encouraged to consult Hill and Rossi (2017).

Reflection question: What wisdom could a client's body send, and how could you help them to get and use that information in one session?

_____

_____

_____

_____

_____

_____

_____

- Milton Erickson is widely recognized as an extraordinarily innovative and effective clinician, a master therapist nonpareil, well known for his brief and effective treatments. He designed specific interventions for different clients. He sent them looking for answers up a local mountain or to a botanical garden, told them metaphorical stories, directed behaviors that would disrupt problems, sometimes had them do the very symptoms they sought to overcome, often used hypnotic trance, and generally practiced therapy in a highly creative way. The basic Ericksonian footprint was described by Steve Lankton (2001) as *matching, blending, utilizing, elaborating ambiguity, reframing,* and *co-creating outcomes.* In 2005, Dan Short, Betty Alice Erickson, and Roxanna Erickson Klein (two of Erickson's daughters) articulated six core Ericksonian strategies: *distraction, partitioning, progression, suggestion, reorientation,* and *utilization.* In 2021, Short set forth six Ericksonian core competencies: *destabilization, naturalistic, strategic, utilization, experiential,* and *tailoring.* Each Erickson case was individualized to fit the particular client. He said: "I wish that Rogerian therapists, Gestalt therapists, transactional group analysts, and all the others would recognize that therapy for person #1 is not psychotherapy for person #2" (quoted in Zeig, 1980, frontispiece). For more about Erickson's professional and personal life, see Zeig (2022a, 2022b).

Erickson sought to use clients' own resources to overcome their problems:

> The fullest possible utilization of the functional capacities and abilities and the experiential and acquisitional learnings of the patient [...] should take precedence over the teaching of new ways in living which are developed from the therapist's possibly incomplete understanding of what may be right and serviceable to the individual concerned.
>
> (Erickson, 1980, p. 540)

✓   One session (SST) was for Erickson the most common length of treatment. In 1990, Bill O'Hanlon and Angela Hexum published *An Uncommon Casebook: The Complete Clinical Work of Milton H. Erickson, M.D.*[8] It contains summaries of many successful SSTs with problems as varied as compulsive thumb-sucking, urinary difficulties, alcohol abuse, intolerance of bright sunlight, cigarette smoking, sexual inhibition and impotence, chronic pain, hiccups, body dysmorphia, marital conflicts, depression, fainting at the sight of blood, phobias, social isolation, and reckless driving. In a page or two, each case is described in terms of the presenting complaint, how long the problem had existed, treatment length and results, and techniques that were used. It's a veritable encyclopedia of brilliant therapy.

✓   In the videotape, *Milton H. Erickson, M.D.: Explorer in Hypnosis and Therapy* (Haley & Richeport, 1993), we learn about his life and see video excerpts of him working successfully in one session with various clients – including a woman ("Monde") who had been abused as a child, and another who was suffering from end-stage cancer and was happy to learn a method to refocus her attention away from the pain. In another, he meets with a young woman ("Nichole") sitting in a wheelchair who became paraplegic as a result of an automobile accident. Erickson, who had post-polio syndrome, is also sitting in a wheelchair. When he asks her what she would like him to do for her, she looks with pleading eyes and says, "Help me walk again." It's quite poignant, the young woman in her chair and the old man in his. He pauses, then asks "And if not that, then what?"

---

8   The title is an allusion to Haley's (1973) *Uncommon Therapy: The Psychiatric Techniques of Milton H. Erickson, M.D.*, the book that introduced Erickson to the wider professional audience. The subtitle of O'Hanlon's (1999) book, *Do One Thing Different: And Other Uncommonly Sensible Solutions to Life's Persistent Problems*, is also an apparent allusion to Haley's (1973) *Uncommon Therapy*. It might be noted that O'Hanlon studied with Erickson and even served for some time as Erickson's gardener; indeed, he wrote a grateful song about Erickson called "Tranceplants" (O'Hanlon, 1996).

(This is what I would call "negotiating a realistic treatment goal" since he isn't able to repair her damaged spinal column.) When she says "Help with my pain," he uses hypnosis and strategic suggestions to get her to better use the muscles she does control. In a 22-year follow-up (Frykman, 2001), we learn that this single session was a turning point for her – she has a full life: married, children, and owns a business.

✓ Another case (reported in O'Hanlon, 1999), known as the "African Violet Queen" involved a lonely and isolated woman living in Milwaukee, Wisconsin, whose apartment was almost lifeless except for being filled with African Violets. She prided herself on her plant collection. Recognizing her Christian belief in kindness and charity, Erickson challenged her to not selfishly keep the lovely plants all to herself but rather to send one as a gift whenever there was a notice in the local newspapers about a bereavement, a graduation, etc. Years later, when the lady passed away, the local newspaper announced, "African Violet Queen Dies – Thousands Mourn." Erickson had utilized her Christian values and horticultural interest to reintegrate her into human society.

✓ At the end of *Uncommon Therapy*, Haley (1973, pp. 270–273) also reported an SST case in which, when all else had failed, Erickson used successfully what Haley described as "an unusual therapeutic strategy," seemingly cruel taunts to stir a post-stroke patient out of a deep funk. On the very last page of the book, however, Haley also writes that Erickson reported that the same patient years later had another debilitating stroke that had rendered him "helpless," and that when the wife asked Erickson to again see the patient, Erickson – knowing his limitations – declined: "I told her I didn't think there was anything more I could do."

✓ In the cases he did attempt, Erickson did not always succeed. Indeed, in the O'Hanlon and Hexum (1990) compendium of 316 cases, there are 15 that they classified as "failures." Some involved men, some women; some individuals and some couples; some were 1–2 sessions, some of unknown duration. In these unsuccessful cases, perhaps it was a lack of psychologically binding conditions and an absence of high emotional tension that kept Erickson from being able to galvanize the patients and help them to move forward (see Rossi, 1973). Erickson (1965, p. 254) looked to himself to make something happen but also included the client's motivations and effort in his search: "Why this is so seems best explained in terms of either the therapist's lack of understanding or the patient's own purposes." It's good to have positive examples for inspiration and instruction, of course, but as I wrote (2000c, p. 193) in "What Can We Learn from Milton Erickson's Therapeutic Failures?": "I find it encouraging to know that even 'The Master' did not hit a home run every time."

Reflection question: Thinking about the Context of Competence described in Chapter 2 (see p. 29), how might you help a client, perhaps in a single session, to utilize their resources to achieve their therapy goals?

_____

_____

_____

_____

_____

_____

_____

- Michele Ritterman (2014) notes that Erickson (in Cooper & Erickson, 1959, p. 247) wrote: "[S]ometimes brief psychotherapy can be remarkably effective [...and] the concept of time distortion lends itself in a remarkable way to clinical therapeutic work." She describes several SST cases in which she assisted clients to overcome problems by having them alter their sense of time (a "fast new stance using the slo-mo three-minute trance") to pinpoint and modify exactly when and how the person's specific problem occurs. In another SST case report (Ritterman, 2005, pp. 2–3; 2019), she describes working with a Central American woman who, pregnant and abandoned by her husband, was feeling desperate / suicidal because of considering having an abortion. Appreciating the woman's social and religious context, Ritterman helps her by appealing to the woman's Catholic beliefs in God and the sanctity of life – the same system of values and beliefs that made the woman feel terrible was utilized as a resource to help her overcome her guilt. Ritterman notes (2019, p. 166) that

> Although many have emphasized Erickson's skills at helping people go into trance, I found Erickson was as much about helping a person do what I call 'Breaking the Spell of a Dysfunctional Rapport' (Ritterman, 1985), that is, helping the person to wake up from a destructive trance.

She also reports (2019, p. 167) an instructive episode seeing Milton Erickson (who was one of her mentors) take a phone call and refuse to see a very overweight person calling for help with weight loss until the person began to lose weight. It was a way of increasing client motivation and also to screen out someone not willing to do anything to bring about the change they ostensibly sought. She recalls what another mentor, Braulio Montalvo, had said, that "the great clinician rejects the impossible cases at the phone call." She (p. 167) explains:

> Erickson was telling this woman that she needed to take charge of the situation herself if she was to receive help from him. [...] His interest was to convey there wouldn't be a minute of that with him. 'Don't waste MY time.' Really also meaning 'Stop wasting YOUR time; and don't call me until you do.' He left the door open.

Reflection question: How might you (maybe in an SST) help a client awaken from a dysfunctional trance?

_____

_____

_____

_____

_____

_____

_____

_____

_____

- Steve Andreas (2014) provides two examples (with transcripts) of SST using neurolinguistic programming (NLP). In one, he assists "Lori" to resolve a phobia and intrusive flashback memories by guiding her to observe the trauma (falling into a bee's nest and getting stung hundreds of times when she was 11 years old) from "outside" rather than from "inside" the experience. He directs her to picture herself in a movie theater projection booth with a glass window between her and a black-and-white image of a bee on the screen. He then gradually has her "run" a tape of the image, gradually changing speeds and switching to color and having her even run the tape backward, over and over. In a few minutes, when he gestures with one finger like a bee coming at Lori, she is momentarily worried, but soon is laughing and reports no longer being fearful. In his discussion, he emphasizes how reactions can be modified by changing how one mentally represents the distressing experience. In the second example, in a single session, he assists another woman to transform a troublesome internal voice by helping her to alter the way she was processing (imagining/representing) it. As Andreas explained in *Transforming Negative Self-Talk: Practical, Effective Exercises* (2012b, p. 1):

> Everyone has internal negative self-talk at times; some of us have this internal chatter going on almost all the time. An internal voice may remind us of past failures, sorrows, or disappointments, torture us with criticism or verbal abuse, describe frightening or unpleasant futures, or disturb us in other ways.

He presents a variety of ways to alter these experiences. In my review (Hoyt, 2012, p. 19) of Andreas' book I noted: "I have used some of these exercises both on myself and with clients and they worked well and quickly."

Long ago, William James (1890, p. 293) said, "Each world whilst it is attended to is real after its own fashion." Reviewing Daniel Kahneman's *Thinking, Fast and Slow* (2011), Andreas (2012a, p. 23) wrote:

> When people remember trauma, they typically experience the most intense moment of pain, or they have a short 'movie' that ends with a high intensity of pain. A ridiculously simple and effective intervention is to ask a client to lengthen the scope of their movie of a traumatic memory so that it ends at a time of less intense unpleasantness, and thus is remembered as less disturbing. This experiment and the many others described in the book, present examples of what is called the 'availability heuristic.' The experience of the ending of pain is more *available* than its duration. By changing the ending point, what is available to memory is changed. WYSIATI [What You See Is All There Is]. Anything you can do to change the experience someone thinks of in the problem state will change what is immediately available to his or her awareness, and change the response. A posthypnotic suggestion is one way. Dr. Erickson's use of a startling interruption of an existing problem response, and then redirecting attention to something else is another. As he once said, 'Your task is that of altering, not abolishing.'

Reflection question: How might you in a single session help a client to imagine themselves distant from and moved beyond the experience and impact of a painful past event?

_____

_____

_____

_____

_____

_____

_____

- Don Meichenbaum (in Hoyt, 1996/2001e, p. 104) also emphasizes that there is more to the story, that we should help the client to not stop at the worst point:

> As the radio commentator Paul Harvey highlights, there is a need to hear 'the rest of the story.' Clients come in and tell their stories. Their stories are often filled with expressions of hopelessness and helplessness. They often convey a tale of having been victimized by individuals, by events, by their feelings and thoughts. It is my job, as the therapist, to not only hear their stories and empathize with them, but also to help them appreciate what they have done to survive and to cope with their feelings – namely, help them attend to 'the rest of the story.' For 'the rest of the story' is often the tale of remarkable strengths. [...] There are a number of clinical techniques designed to accomplish this goal and to incorporate these features into their personal narratives. Thus, the 'bad things' that happened to people are only one chapter in their life stories. And, as Judith Herman (1992) indicates, it is *not* the most interesting chapter of their autobiographies.

In her book *The Therapeutic "Aha!": Strategies for Getting Your Clients Unstuck*, Courtney Armstrong (2015, pp. 111–113) similarly advises:

> Stories generally have a beginning, middle, and end. But when it comes to traumatic memories, the mind tends to end the story as the worst moment or leave the story unfinished. Thus, to resolve a traumatic memory, assist the client in finishing the story at a place where

he escaped, recovered, or had a more pleasant encounter later in his life. The ending of a story doesn't necessarily have to be happy, just useful.

She notes that Odysseus returns from his hero's journey wiser and reunites with his family, and "the Tin Man finds his heart and the Lion discovers his courage." The wounded warrior persists. The beat goes on. Continuing the story might involve considering a traumatic memory as a prolonged fermata, a "long pause" (hyphen) rather than a "full stop" (period), so to speak. This "re-punctuating" might occur in a single session, helping the client to get "unstuck" and to move forward.[9]

Meichenbaum (2012, p. 3) defines *resilience* as "the capacity to adapt successfully to the presence of risk and adversity," and he and George Bonanno (2021) present clear evidence and describe methods – sometimes applicable in a single session – to contradict the idea that most people get permanently damaged by stressful events. Although some will develop problems such as PTSD, depression, and substance abuse, after trauma most people use flexible strategies to cope and recover. In *Roadmap to Resilience: A Guide for Military, Trauma Victims and Their Families*, Meichenbaum (2012) describes six areas (each with specific potential actions, useful information, and inspiring quotable quotes) in which post-traumatic coping and growth can be enhanced:

✓ Physical fitness
✓ Interpersonal fitness
✓ Emotional fitness
✓ Thinking (cognitive) fitness
✓ Behavioral fitness
✓ Spiritual fitness

---

9 An interesting variant of extending the story was described to me by Michele Ritterman (personal communication, February 18, 2024), who adapted a technique she learned from her mentor, Milton Erickson. Working with a client who was very anxious about an upcoming cardiac procedure that required no consuming food after midnight the night before, she asked about what food the person would have to break the fast afterwards. The person started musing about pizza (what toppings?) versus French fries (regular or garlic?) versus chocolates (milk or dark?), etc., etc. The food fantasies had captured his imagination (rather than the medical woes) – and then he realized that "*after* the procedure" meant he would survive, and his angst greatly diminished.

Reflection question: How might you in a single session help a client to improve their resilience and perhaps experience post-traumatic growth?

_____

_____

_____

_____

_____

_____

_____

_____

- Robert Kellner, Joseph Neidhardt, Barry Krakow, and Diane Pathak (1992) report two single session treatments effective for ameliorating chronic recurring nightmares. In one, they have the client describe their nightmare, teach the client progressive muscle relaxation (PMR), and then have the client develop an exposure hierarchy and work their way through the hierarchy while practicing relaxation – an application of systematic desensitization (Wolpe, 1958) in which anxiety and relaxation are mutually incompatible. In the other condition, the researchers would hear about the nightmare and teach the client PMR, and then in the relaxed state have the client imagine a new, happy ending to the nightmare story. For both conditions, there was the single session in the office and clients were then instructed to practice twice a day for two weeks. Both conditions were helpful – for both, at 7-month follow-up, there was a significant decrease in the frequency of nightmares and marked improvement on self-rated questionnaires of anxiety and depression. To maximize compliance and benefit, I have found it useful to

(a) describe both treatments to a client ("A study was done at the University of New Mexico in which they developed two effective treatments for nightmares like yours. In one condition, they taught the people to relax and then to gradually think about the nightmare while staying relaxed; in the other condition they taught the people to relax and when relaxed had them think of and rehearse a new ending so that the nightmare would no longer bother them – which would be better for you?") and then ask the client to pick the one they feel will be best for them (which promotes positive expectations and buy-in; most people choose the new ending);

(b) provide the client with a copy of the original Kellner et al. report (or a brief written summary), to provide information for informed consent and to enhance clinician credibility; and

(c) have the client take home a copy of the journal research article (or summary) as a reminder of both the treatment and the therapist (a talisman and transitional object).

Additionally, as Goldfield and Hoyt (2022) report, while clients are in a relaxed state from doing the PMR, they can be given suggestions to enhance the desired positive outcome.

Reflection question: How might you adapt this in a single session to a variety of worries, not just nightmares?

_____

_____

_____

_____

_____

_____

_____

_____

• Michael Yapko (1990a) provides a full transcript of a single-session hypnotherapy done with a 42-year-old woman ("Vicki") who was referred for help in coping with terminal cancer.[10] First interviewing the patient in a conversational manner, he builds rapport while identifying treatment goals, potential pitfalls, and various resources – which are then

---

10 In the fourth edition of his opus magnum, *Trancework: An Introduction to the Practice of Clinical Hypnosis,* Yapko (2012) provides a DVD of the entire session with Vicki. As he writes in the book (2012, p. 512): "This session is as dramatic as sessions can be, with life and death literally hanging in the balance." He goes on: "You may notice something else: I never used the word *pain* during our session, even though that's why she was there. The word pain has a strong negative emotional attachment to it, for it represents both a physical condition and an emotionally charged experience that is most unpleasant. Use of the word pain, therefore, should be avoided whenever possible. You can substitute less charged words like *pressure, discomfort,* or *uncomfortable sensation* in place of the word pain." Battino (2010, 2020) also advises carefully using language that is healing rather than hurtful.

utilized in the second portion of the SST, which involves more formal hypnotic induction and trancework. Suggestions are made to facilitate dissociation, time distortion, appetite enhancement, alteration in kinesthetic awareness, and reframing of uncertainty as being pleasant in order to help her reduce emotional distress and physical discomfort. We learn that the SST was very helpful until her physical condition became too severe to self-manage.

Reflection question: When someone is in pain and facing end of life, what can a psychotherapist do (maybe in one session) to help them?

- Gregory Walton and Geoffrey Cohen (2011) describe a one-session social-belonging intervention to improve academic and health outcomes of minority students. They got them to write a little essay about how feelings of not belonging are temporary and normal for a while but that the feelings change and the person becomes more comfortable over time. Follow-up at three years showed significant improvement in grade point averages, academic achievement, and health measures. This performance boost was interpreted as mediated by the effect of the intervention on subjective construal: It prevented students from seeing adversity on campus as an indictment of their belonging. While these findings were especially true for African American students (who were more subject to stereotyping and marginalization), the social-belonging intervention could also be used with others who may have a less-than-secure sense of belonging (e.g., persons who are the first in their family to attend college or those who are entering new, previously restricted fields).

Reflection question: How in an SST might someone benefit from being helped to perceive their sense of disconnection as temporary and passing?

_____
_____
_____
_____
_____
_____
_____
_____
_____

- David Feldman and Diane Dreher (2012) conducted a test of the efficacy of a single session 90-minute goal-pursuit intervention for college students. Hope involves the belief that there's a way to get there and that it can be done (Frank, 1968; Snyder, 2002; Courtnage, 2020; Hoyt, 2021). They had college students first identify a specific goal and then describe and articulate the small, particular steps they would take to achieve the goal. Focusing on operationalizing instrumentality, on having the students break down the task into do-able parts, in one session hope and subsequent actual goal attainment were enhanced compared to control subjects.

Reflection question: What does the old joke "Q. How do you eat an elephant? A. One bite at a time!" mean? (Hint: The epigraph, that opens this book, from Lao Tzu in the 6th century BCE, says: "The journey of a thousand miles begins with a single step.") How might this be applied in an SST?

_____
_____
_____
_____
_____
_____
_____
_____
_____

- There are many other examples of SST that could be cited. To mention a few that may have special interest (also see Appendix A):

✓ Single-session sex therapy (Springmann, 1978; Flemons & Green, 2014)

✓ Equine-assisted single session consultations (Green, 2014) and group-administered single-session canine therapy (Binfet, 2017)

✓ Single session therapy for those affected by gambling (Cohen, Daley, & Northe, 2021; Rodda, Lubman, Cheetham, Dowling, & Jackson, 2015; Rodda, Lubman, Jackson, & Dowling, 2017; Tolchard, Thomas, & Battersby, 2006)

✓ Single session music therapy with people who are chemically dependent (Jones, 2005)

✓ Successful one-session resolution of auditory hallucinations (Blymyer, 1991)

✓ One-session resolution of an hysterical symptom (Oremland, 1976)

✓ Single session therapy to help clients reduce high-risk sexual behavior (Dilley, Woods, Loeb, Nelson, Sheon, Mullan, et al., 2007; Dilley, Woods, Sabatino, Lihatsh, Adler, Casey, S., et al., 2002; Buttram, Kurtz, & Surratt, 2013; Sagherian, Huedo-Medina, Pellowski, Eaton, & Johnson, 2016; Loughlin, 2021)

✓ Inpatient psychiatric groups ("I believe that the inpatient group therapist must consider the life of the group to be only a single session" – Yalom & Leszcz, 2005, p. 488)

✓ Single session dance/movement therapy for people with acute schizophrenia (Biondo & Gerber, 2020)

✓ Single Session Therapy to reduce self-harm (Cowmesadow, 1995; Lamprecht, Laydon, McQuillan, Wiseman, Williams, Gash, & Reilly, 2007)

✓ Single session vocational counseling (Barrett, Lapsley, & Agee, 2012)

✓ Single session "dreamscaping" for grief and loss (Gershman & Thompson, 2019)

✓ SST delivered via the Internet (Babling et al., 2008; Rodda et al., 2015; Rodda et al., 2017; Ziadni, Gonzalez-Castro, Anderson, Krishnamurthy, & Darnall, 2021; Bennett et al., 2022; Dryden, in press; Hartley et al., 2023; Moore et al., in press; Slive & Bobele, in press; Schleider, 2024; van Empel, 2024, in press)

✓ There are also various protocols and programs offering structured one-session processes for stress reduction, smoking cessation, pain management, and improved sleep

✓ Many visits to a medical doctor or dentist are also essentially single sessions – there is one meeting in which a problem is identified and a treatment provided (sometimes involving medication to be taken after the session). It is a one-off; the patient returns on an as-needed basis.

The many examples presented here, drawn from SST experts using a variety of theoretical approaches and involving a panoply of SST principles and practices, are offered to "plant seeds" and to "open doors." Some of the ideas and methods may already be familiar; some may add to your therapeutic repertoire. Readers are encouraged to adapt and apply as appropriate.

In the following chapter, we will continue to examine SST case examples to see what useful lessons can be garnered, now turning to ones from my own practice.

SST Examples from My Practice

5

Here, we will consider some SST examples drawn from my own experience – most as a therapist, two as a client – and then conclude with some more general reflections. Each example is offered as a springboard for consideration of how you might adapt and apply some of the methods in a single session with some of your clients. In addition to the ideas I suggest, please generate your own.

- Hoyt and Talmon (1990) and Hoyt (expanded version, 2000d/2017, pp. 134–152) report my first case from the Kaiser SST study, which I have come to call "The Case of the Intrusive Father." As a videotape of the session shows (see Figure 5.1), the 29-year-old female client sought help to deal with her highly intrusive and inappropriate ne'er-do-well biological father, who had called from the local county jail demanding that she visit and bring him money and cigarettes and candy. She wanted help with both disturbing memories of his behavior during her childhood as well as his current demands and her anxious anticipation of when he would next appear uninvited at her door. In the single session, we looked at possible family models ("How does your aunt deal with him?"), role-played confronting him at the door (we went to the office door and imagined he was there), reviewed lessons she had learned from the experience, and discussed next steps ("When he calls…when he comes to the door").

  In this case and in the following case, I was strongly influenced by my Redecision Therapy training with Mary and Bob Goulding (1979; also see

DOI: 10.4324/9781003468547-5

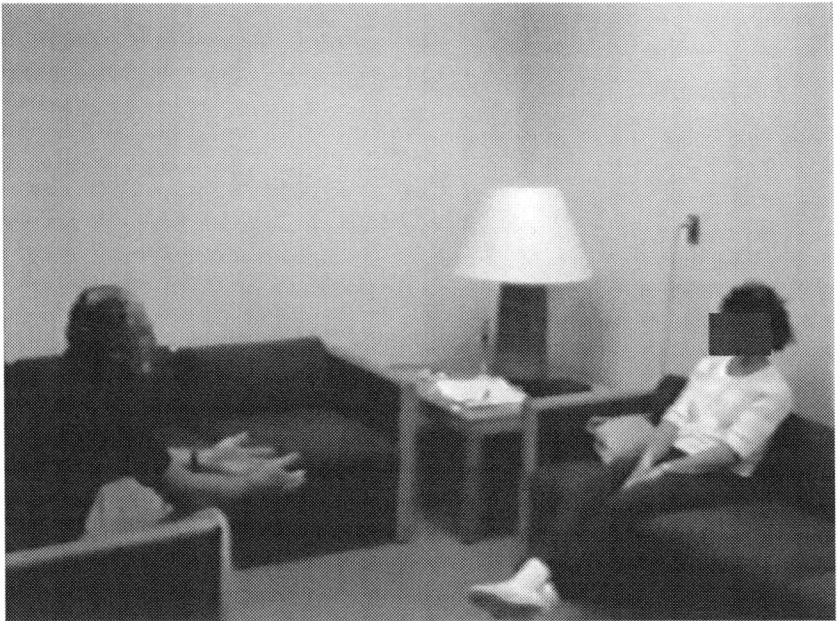

Figure 5.1 The First Minute of My First SST Session in the Kaiser Research Project, Circa 1987 (screen shot from video).

Source: ©M.F. Hoyt 2018. Used with permission.

Hoyt & Goulding, 1989/1995; Hoyt, 1995/2001; and discussion of Gouldings' Redecision model and case of "Anne" presented above in Chapter 4 on p. 90), who advocated having clients enact/role-play desired changes (not just talk about them) to help reify the changes. This is consistent with both Milton Erickson's advice (in Zeig, 1980, p. 72; also see Zeig, 2018) that "I believe that patients and students should do things. They learn better, remember better" as well as Carl Whitaker's (1983, p. 400) comment that "Explanation leads to recognition, experience leads to change."

Reflection question: How can you help an SST client to practice a desired solution?

_____

_____

_____

_____

_____

_____

_____

_____

- In Rosenbaum, Hoyt, and Talmon (1990/1995, pp.125–127) and Talmon, Hoyt, and Rosenbaum (1990, pp. 45–47), I recount how a woman who requested a "divorce ceremony" had a single session in which she read a poem she had written, burned a photograph of her father, underwent some guided imagery of her holding and healing her inner child, and then presented and had the therapist and her husband (as well as herself) sign a "Decree of Divorce" that she had printed on her home computer. A lot happened in one session!

Reflection question: What ceremony, ritual, role-play, in-session enactment, experiential practice activity, etc. could be helpful with one (or more) of your SST clients?

_____

_____

_____

_____

_____

_____

_____

- Hoyt (1994b, pp. 150–150, italics in original) described using an SST to help a client revise her self-image and prepare for subsequent therapy. An attractive but cheaply made-up young woman was on her way out of town, "headed for a new life" she said. She had been working as an "exotic dancer" at a local adult theater, and she told stories that indicated why she had tired of such an existence. Somehow, she had decided to use her health insurance before leaving town and had made an appointment and was in my office. She had no specific goals or agenda, she said, she just wanted to see what the Psychiatry Department might have to offer that could help her. One session might be useful, I thought, to help prepare her for possible subsequent therapeutic work and to make a referral. I complimented her on her desire to find a life that would be more satisfying to her. [...] I asked if she was bright, and she said "Yes, why?" I explained that since we would only have one meeting, I wanted to say something that would make more sense to a bright person. She nodded, and I said,

> Have you ever seen a really bad bruise? You know, one that aches and turns yellow and green? I work here in a medical center so I see such things. Well, anyway, from what you've told me, I think that in some ways you've been bruised psychologically, from what you've been through. But from what you've told me I can also tell that *nothing is broken, that all the bruises can heal.* Know what I mean?

She nodded again, and one could almost see her self-image revising, from "broken" to "bruised," from "ruined" to "repairable." I went on to suggest that she might want to get into therapy once she relocated, "when you're ready,"[1] and suggested that it would be good for her to have someone she could get to know and depend on over time. I gave her the names of two counseling centers in the town she was planning to move to. Almost a year later, I got a call from a therapist in another town. Our patient had changed her plans and had relocated in a different area. She was now in therapy.

In another case (reported in Hoyt & Battino, 2022), "Joey" was a bright college student whose parents dragged him into my office because of their concerns about his frequent use of cannabis. He had agreed, reluctantly, to come for one session. Their worries about his grades going down and his increasingly unpleasant mood were met with, "It's legal in California, so what's the problem?" As I watched, all anti-drug arguments they voiced were anticipated and quickly batted aside. When they finally looked toward me, rather than quoting the usual (and probably expected) shaming slogan, "Drugs are for people who can't handle reality," I said: *"Reality is for people who can't handle drugs."* Joey looked confused: "Huh?" I waited a bit, letting it hang in the air, then replied: "The part of you that's smart heard me. Whatchathink?" This led into

---

1   As said Shakespeare (*Hamlet*, Act V, Scene II, lines 234–237):

> If it be now, 'tis not to come;
> if it be not to come, it will be now;
> if it be not now, yet it will come.
> The readiness is all.

a nuanced discussion about use versus abuse. Joey acknowledged his "overuse" (his term), and we began to discuss what Joey would need to do differently. He subsequently made an appointment with a counselor on the Chemical Dependency Team.

In the case of the "exotic dancer," she was very invested in her appearance so I used the metaphor of bruises; when a young hippie fellow came in wearing a Grateful Dead tee-shirt, I said (Hoyt, 2009b, p. 9) "What a long strange trip it's been, huh?" With Joey, I appealed to his intelligence, said something unexpected, and treated him respectfully.

Reflection questions: (1) If it seems unlikely that one session will be adequate for the client to make the changes they desire, what would be useful for the SST? and (2) Is there something about the client that suggests a way to speak with her or him that will register?

_____

_____

_____

_____

_____

_____

_____

_____

- As reported in Hoyt and Battino (2021), "Ned" was a fellow in his 40s when I first met him. For years, he would contact me sporadically – usually for one visit, sometimes for two. He often spent days driving around buying and selling junk without making much profit. He was friendly but seemed "eccentric" and was living a marginal existence: low-income housing, no steady work, or consistent romantic partner. (His therapy copayment was covered by state welfare insurance.) We met when he wanted to discuss a concern, such as his father's failing health or his brother's addictions and demands, or sometimes when he just wanted "to check in." There was never a specific desired "change" outcome from a session – just "I want to come and talk with you."

We enjoyed our visits, but I wasn't sure how useful or "therapeutic" they were. But when I was getting ready to retire from the clinic, he heard that I was leaving and requested an appointment. When we met, he thanked me for being "very supportive" and "having been there" for him over the years. He said that he always left our meetings encouraged and felt appreciated and affirmed rather than being dismissed as just another "do-nothing weirdo" (his term).

I don't think that SST "failed" to help Ned. Although most of us therapists may conceive of ourselves as being agents of change, it is our client's right to not change. Ned sought – and received – support and human connection.

Reflection questions: Are there clients you know who might benefit in a single session simply by being able to "check in"? How might they indicate that?

_____

_____

_____

_____

_____

_____

_____

_____

• Hoyt and Insoo Kim Berg (1998) discuss the solution-focused brief therapy videotape depicting Berg (1994) working with a struggling couple ("Bill and Leslie"). Insoo keeps her eye on the prize, pleasantly and persistently staying focused on where the clients want to go and not getting sucked into their arguments and bickering. She keeps her sail out of their wind, figuratively speaking, unless it's blowing in the direction they really want to go. As my then 11-year-old son said after watching portions of the videotape: "Dad, that's good. Instead of letting them fight, she's getting them to talk about ways they could be happier." In workshops, I have sometimes shown the entire session and have the audience break into "problem detectives" and "solution detectives" (Sharry, Madden, & Darmody, 2001) – each side looking for problems/weaknesses versus strengths/resources and then comparing notes. As de Shazer (1985, p. 7, italics in original) wrote:

> For an intervention to successfully *fit*, it is not necessary to have detailed knowledge of the complaint. it is not necessary even to be able to construct with any rigor how the trouble is maintained in order to prompt solution. [...] *any* really different behavior in a problematic

situation can be enough to prompt solution and give the client the satisfaction he [or she] seeks from therapy.

Reflection questions: How can you help clients to stay focused on their desired goal? Suppose a "miracle happened" and after the SST your client began to achieve more of what they had sought therapy for – what might be the first things you and they would notice are different? And then what?

- Hoyt (1994b) and Hoyt and Cannistrà (2023a, pp. 130–131) present examples of single-session SFBT with couples. In both cases, the work is quite straightforward, involving:

  ✓ Asking the Miracle Question: "Suppose tonight, while you're sleeping, a miracle happens, and the problems that brought you here are resolved. Tomorrow, when you wake up, how will you notice that the miracle has occurred?"
  ✓ Some prompting and probing to help them talk about good times, past and future, in order to get them to see each other again as sources of light (not darkness).
  ✓ Pursuing questions to get details and specific plans for fun and pleasure in order to rekindle hope and help them shift from a problem-saturated story (White & Epston, 1990) to a more hopeful solution-oriented narrative (Hudson & O'Hanlon, 1992; Weiner-Davis, 1992; Hoyt, 2015).

In both cases, by the end of the respective single sessions, the couples were feeling happy, had skills, plans, and motivation ready, and did not think that another appointment would be necessary but agreed to call back as needed.

I'm in favor of "divorce busting" (Weiner-Davis, 1992) but, if at the end of a single session a couple decided not to work on saving their marriage, I would not necessarily consider that to be a bad outcome. Cannistrà (in Torricelli, 2021, p. 139) makes a similar observation: "Couple's therapy does not always end with the rapprochement of partners." In a chapter about SST/OAAT couple therapy titled "Change or Not – That is the Question," Söderquist (2023, p. 18) also describes a session in which it was at first unclear whether the couple will continue their relationship:

> Both turn to each other and simultaneously and laughingly they say: 'separation.' This was very unexpected to me, and I can just say: 'Are we where you wanted to be in the session?' They both agree. We continue the session with a discussion and their plans for how to do the separation. They seem to be in agreement and relieved.

Comment: In my experience, most affairs/infidelity issues aren't going to get resolved in one session – acknowledgment, apologies, anger, rebuilding trust, disappointment, more anger, more apologies, more rebuilding trust, dealing with the ex-lover (who may be in the workplace), etc. There are also different kinds of affairs – one-nighters, repeated promiscuity (sometimes sex addiction), an ongoing deep emotional as well as physical connection, etc. In a first (only?) session, I think a couple needs to walk out with hope, motivation to save the marriage, and something of a plan – otherwise, why come in and (maybe) why come back? Each case is different, of course, but I would want to clarify "What do you want to get from today's meeting and from therapy?" We might even do some pros/cons discussion of staying together versus breaking up, possibly with motivational interviewing methods to enhance their hope and wanting to stay together – i.e., having them voice the "pros" for staying. I'd try to get stories about their love. I'd probably also say that there's some hard work ahead and there will be moments they'll want to just give up, but if they can get through it and come out together they'll be stronger (and if kids are involved, remind them that they don't want to damage the kids – divorce isn't good for kids, but neither is living in a house full of anger and hate). I once suggested to a man that he go on Sunday morning to the local pancake restaurant to see all the fathers and unhappy kids finishing their weekend visitation – since that was where they were likely heading if he didn't change what he was doing. He did go and it motivated him to clean up his act. Sometimes, it helps to have a couple read a book. It gives them a roadmap, lets them know others have been through this, and that it is something they can do together. If you Google "books on recovering from affairs," you'll see that there are a lot available. I wouldn't recommend anything to a couple, however, unless I've read it myself – just to make sure it's appropriate, that there won't be something in it that will cause more trouble, etc.

A couple sought an appointment. When we sat down and I asked, "What are you hoping for from our meeting today?" the woman replied, "Like the old newspaper column used to ask, 'Can this marriage be saved?'" I responded, "Maybe. That's not up to me. That will depend on what you're willing to do." Despite my many efforts to look for hopes and exceptions, after 45 minutes of hearing about a nasty bilateral lack of respect, long-time alienation of affection, repeated infidelities on both sides, and a mutual unwillingness to take responsibility for problems or solutions ("No, SHE's / HE's the one that needs to change!") I looked at the clock and said, "We only have a few minutes left today – should we make another appointment? What do you think?" The woman replied: "I don't think so. We already have an appointment with a divorce law-yer, but just wanted to give counseling a chance."

Reflection question: Did we stop too soon? If the clients don't want to continue, when should you try to "hold 'em and when should you fold 'em"?

_____

_____

_____

_____

_____

_____

_____

_____

- Hoyt (2004) reports a one-hour clinical demonstration interview done at the 1998 Brief Therapy: Lasting Impressions conference held in New York City. A man volunteered who was dealing with multiple stresses: his mother had recently died, his young daughter was facing a major, nine-hour surgery; the man struggled with "not-good-enough" self-esteem problems and had chronic difficulty relaxing; and in the background, there lurked issues having to do with conflicts between his parents and the way his father had treated him when young. Some notable features of the interview include:

✓ At the beginning, the way the therapist needed to move from a global "What's up?" to a more targeted "How can I help you today – what do you want to change?"

✓ Use of hopeful, suppositional language (*"After* the surgery, *when* things are better, what will..."* – rather than *"if* things are better...")

✓ The use of the narrative therapy (White & Epston, 1990) methods of *personification* and *externalization and relative influence questioning* ("What do you call this pressure? Does it have a name? When is it in charge of you and when are you in charge of it? What's the difference?"). Some exploration of the history with his father of his self-esteem / negative self-talk issues, with an emphasis on how the client can resist negative messages.

✓ When the client reveals that when, as a child he had a sister who underwent a serious surgery and did not survive, the therapist encourages rationality (p. 38): "How do you remind yourself that your sister's not your daughter, that what happened with your sister doesn't mean anything in terms of the outcome for your daughter?"

✓ Emphasis on coping strategies that the client can use during the stressful waiting-for-daughter's-surgery period, including reading, time with wife and friends, and evoking the late mother as an ally (e.g., "Do you think your mom would be glad to see you taking more time?")

✓ Future-pacing of desired changes (e.g., "When you make some of these changes now and into the next months, who else is going to help you with that?")

✓ In the termination phase of the session, the therapist encourages lexical encoding (putting it into words) to help the client conceptualize and store ideas or lessons in a retrievable way (e.g., "In a couple of minutes we'll stop, but I wanted to ask you before we stop – what's been helpful in our talking? What's something you'll carry with you?") In response to the client's expressed desire to stay more present-focused (rather than worrying about the future), the therapist offers a catchy refrain to help the client recall a learning when the pressure's on: "Yesterday is history and tomorrow's a mystery, today is a gift, and that's why they call it the present." A well-targeted joke, song lyric, or memorable image might similarly be a useful mnemonic or anchor (see Beaulieu, 2004; Hoyt & Andreas, 2015).

When working with a client who presents with multiple stressful issues, the therapist can decide which issue to focus on (usually one that is immediate and likely to be helped, like assisting the client described above to cope with anxiety while waiting for his daughter's surgery so that the client can have a successful experience and feel encouraged); but it may be even better to ask the client (for example), "Given all that you've got going on – your mom, your daughter, your difficulties with relaxing and feeling OK, stuff with your father – which issue do YOU think we should address today?" Allowing the *client* to choose empowers the client and begins to bring order to their sense of being overwhelmed. There's an old saying, "If you're too well rounded, you're not pointed in any direction." So, how to proceed?

Reflection question: How do you and the client *figure out how and what to be focused on (prioritization, treatment planning) rather than just trying to cover everything all at once?*

_____

_____

_____

_____

_____

_____

_____

- As reported in Hoyt (2009c), Sam was a 67-year-old man when I first met him sitting in a wheelchair next to his wife in the waiting room of the HMO Psychiatry clinic. He had been referred by his internist: "Post-stroke. Fear of falling." When I introduced myself and we shook hands, I could see that he was a pleasant and engaging man. He had not shaved in a few days, was casually dressed, and was wearing an Oakland A's baseball cap. His wife immediately began to talk (a lot) and quickly told me that Sam could walk but was afraid to. He had come into the building on his own, and then gotten into the wheelchair. She was nice and trying to be helpful, but I sensed that it would be useful to have some time with the patient alone, so I asked: "Do you want to walk or ride to my office?" He replied: "I'll take a ride, at least this time."

  As I pushed him around the corner and down the corridor, we talked baseball – about a recent trade and how the game had gone that day.

Knowing that the star player had batted 2-for-4 and his average went up six points and what the manager had said after the game seemed more vital than being able to count backward by 7's or recite the names of presidents. His remarks showed a good knowledge and alert, up-to-date interest. I asked questions, and we connected as we talked.

At my office door, I stopped and asked if he could take a few steps into my office and use a regular chair, so that I would not have to move the furniture around – an indirect approach that used his natural courtesy to bypass discussion of his need for the wheelchair. He obliged. When we sat down, I learned that he was a retired mechanic and printing press-man. He had suffered a stroke three years earlier, with a residual partial paralysis of one arm and leg. He had grown "too damn dependent" on his wife, he said, but could no longer drive and had considerable difficulty walking. "I sure miss Dr. Jarrett," he interjected, referring to his former internist who had himself retired a few years earlier. I asked what Dr. Jar-rett would have said to get him moving. When he told me, I "borrowed" the good doctor's mantle of authority and replied: "Took the words right out of my mouth."

Sam went on to tell me that he wanted to go to an upcoming game his sons had invited him to, but he had to first overcome his great fear of fall-ing because "I get so worried and down that I freeze up." He knew how to fall safely (protecting his head and softening the fall) but was fearful because "I'm not sure what would happen to me if I fell and no one was around. I might not be able to get back up."

(By coincidence, I had the night before read my then young son a story [Peet, 1972] about a series of animals that each gets stranded, culminating with an elephant stuck on his back until an ant he had befriended rescues him with the help of an ant hoard.)

Sam was a practical man with a predicament. After ascertaining that he was not worried about safety or embarrassment, I suggested: "I'll tell you what. Let's do a little experiment. I'll be you, you be the coach, and teach me how to get up." I then proceeded to sort of throw myself on the floor in front of him. He got right into it, advising me, "No, turn the other way, get up first on three points," etc. I said, "Let's try it with my arm not working" and held it limply (post-stroke like) against my side. For the next several minutes, I repeatedly got down on the floor and Sam instructed me on how to get myself up again.

Back in my chair, I asked him if he wanted to "try it" there in my office or wait until he got home – an "illusion of alternatives" (Watzlawick, 1978) with the underlying implication that he would perform the action. He chose to wait until he was home but offered to show me "some exercises I can still do." I watched and then asked him to "stand and do a little walking just so I can see how you do." I opened the office door and we proceeded into the corridor. We slowly made our way up and down the hallway, with my remarking a couple of times "Good" and "Nice, better than I expected." As we went up and down the hallway, I switched back to baseball, asking him about the game he was planning to attend with his sons. "Where are you going to park? Which ramp will you take?" I painted aloud a vivid picture of father and sons entering the baseball stadium as we made our way up and down the hallway a couple of times.

Back in my office he expressed concern about his wife. He recognized that she was trying to be helpful but she was wearing out both herself and Sam with her watchfulness. "Maybe you could talk to her, too," he asked. I said I would be glad to "when you begin to do more walking on your own so that I'll really be able to convince her to back off." He understood and agreed to practice his falling and getting up, and we playfully bargained about how many times he would do it a day, settling on twice a day to start and then three times a day until I saw him in two weeks.

Before leaving my office I added,

> You know, I think it's really important that you go to that game with your sons if you can. I know you want to, but I think it will be even more important for them. Someday they will look back and remember going to the game with you, you know what I mean?

Sam did not know exactly how baseball was in my blood, my history of going to games with my father, but he knew I was saying something heartfelt and important. It spoke to him. "I'm sure going to give it my best," he said. "Dr. Jarrett would like that," I replied.

When next I saw Sam he proudly walked into my office, slowly. He had been practicing and was eagerly anticipating going to the game the next week with his sons. I then brought his wife into the session and we talked about ways she could help by doing things and ways she could help by not doing things. Two weeks later, he told me about going to the game and his plans to go to another one. He also expressed the desire for more activity, and I suggested attending an Older Adults Therapy Group as well as some other outings with neighbors and former coworkers. He followed through on these suggestions, and I remained available if and when he might again request to meet with me.

Sam's worries about falling were taken seriously. The approach here was highly pragmatic, strategies being directed toward quickly getting the patient walking. It was helpful and felt natural to temporarily reverse roles, Sam becoming the teacher/coach rather than the humbled stroke patient. This was morale restoring and opened possibilities for change. The hallway walk into the ballpark was hypnotic and future oriented. His desire for assistance in managing his wife was used to further promote treatment compliance. Part of effective brief therapy is deciding what paths *not* to take. Exploring Sam's concerns about failing powers and limited mortality were issues that might be worthwhile (and would be addressed in the Older Adults group), but first helping Sam to regain his confidence in walking and being able to get up when he fell enhanced the quality of his life and put him in a stronger position to realistically appraise his future options. This is what Sam and his wife wanted. Being alert to and using whatever resources are available in the service of the client's therapeutic needs – including the therapist's own personal experiences with baseball, inverted elephants, and father-son relations[2] – is what I take Milton Erickson and Ernest Rossi (1979, p. 276) to mean when they suggest: "To initiate this type of therapy you have to be yourself as a person. You cannot imitate somebody else, but you have to do it your own way."

As I said in Hoyt and Cannistrà (2023, pp. 21–22) when talking about this case:

> So when I was reading this, I had a 'Oh my gosh, the case was 20 years ago!' realization. […] I realized that now I am the same age that he was, actually a couple of years older – oh my gosh! And when I talked to him about his sons, and in the stuff we did in the office, he was an older man and I was a younger man. We had a bit of a father-son relationship. The reason I bring all this up is that the alliance we form with people depends on who we are at a certain time and now when people come to see me they see a grandfather or bald-head or an uncle or older gentleman or something like that, whereas 30 years ago or 20 years ago it was different. It made sense when I saw 'Sam' for him

---

2 I love the story my father told me (recounted in Hoyt, 1995a, pp. 331–332) about the time he was at a baseball game at Wrigley Field in Chicago, and a drunken and belligerent fan in the bleachers was verbally abusing one of the ballplayers. The man let it be known that he was packing a gun, and it became increasingly possible that he might use it. My father – who was a salesman by trade and something of a strategic therapist by nature – got involved. Dad was also a gun fancier; and he got the irate fan engaged in a discussion about the type of gun, showed some interest, and wound up bargaining for and buying the gun on the spot. (The police never came.) When I asked my father what he had done with the weapon, he said he had taken it to a shop the next day and sold it, for a profit. When I asked why he had done that, he replied: "Hey, you've got to get paid for this kind of work!"

to be the wise coach and for him to tell me how to do certain things, because that put him in the senior authority, expert adult role, compared to me. Part of what we did was I playfully threw myself on the floor and Sam repeatedly coached me on how to get up. If I did that with somebody now that would seem strange to them, it would not seem natural. 'Why is this old man falling down on the floor in front of me and asking me how he should get up?' They would probably call 911 or the security guard! [...] You have to think of the therapeutic relationship. You can't just do what's in the book because the book doesn't say 'He's sitting in a wheelchair' (or 'You're sitting in a wheelchair'). People are going to respond to that person differently than to some young, strong, healthy-looking person.

Reflection question: In SST we endeavor to efficiently form an alliance and establish a session goal. How does who you are and who the client is effect how you connect and what options may be available?

_____
_____
_____
_____
_____
_____
_____
_____

• Hoyt and Michele Ritterman (2012) describe a single session of "Brief Therapy in a Taxi." On our way to visit the Erickson house in Phoenix, we got into a discussion with the taxi driver who told us a sad story about how, several years earlier, his wife who he had thought was the love of his life had suddenly abandoned him and had moved to another city. He had felt puzzled and sucker-punched. It got quiet in the taxi.

'Have you heard the one about the taxi driver?' I asked, getting his attention and taking advantage of this moment to make an alternative suggestion that our driver could possibly accept.

'No.'

'Well, he was driving along when the red lights went on behind him, and a cop pulled him over.' The cabbie glanced over his shoulder at the mention of a policeman coming up behind him. 'The driver begged the cop, 'Please don't give me a ticket.'

And the cop said, 'I'll tell you what. If you can tell me a good story, I'll let you go.'

And the taxi driver replied, 'My wife ran off with a cop. When I saw you, I got scared you were him, and that you were bringing her back!''

Our driver now laughed wholeheartedly. Rejection had switched to escape. When we got to the house and I was paying him, the driver said, 'I'm going to remember that story,' and laughed again. In the moment, despite the past, he might not really want her back. I smiled and gave him a $10 tip to help anchor it. As Erickson taught, context and sequence are important for brief intervention to have maximal chance to take hold.

As Erickson (quoted in Gordon & Meyers-Anderson, 1981, p. 29) said: "You need to teach patients to laugh off their griefs and to enjoy their pleasures." I agree and would add: Humor tickles the neurology that holds us stuck. Laughter disrupts a negative trance. With the right tact and timing, a carefully selected joke has a way of getting past "resistance" and sticking in our mind. We can alter a trance state by providing something unexpected. Carl Whitaker (see 1975) said that humor and absurdity were a "way of getting around the corner without tearing down the building." And the great comedian Mort Sahl (1976, p. 23) wrote: "Humor is the ultimate shorthand." Hoyt and Andreas (2015) discuss humor in brief therapy, and Dryden (2017, pp. 186–187) provides some sensible guidelines for the judicious use of humor in SST (and other therapy).

Reflection question: When have you or could you use a joke, a quip, a silly pun, a double entendre, etc. to help a client make a quick shift?

_____

_____

_____

_____

_____

_____

_____

_____

- Hoyt (1994, p. 148; and 2017, p. 61) describes the single session use of an internalized other as an ally. A widower in his late 60s made an appointment. When we met, he explained that, despite the doctors' confidence and assurances, his wife had died while undergoing cardiac surgery. A quiet talk about how sometimes "bad things happen to good people" may have been supportive, but he was not relieved. He missed her, but his mourning and adjustment were being badly tormented by a gnawing sense of painful survivor's guilt. I commented that the experts on guilt are judges and lawyers, and that although we were talking about psychological (not legal) guilt, they tell us that two conditions have to obtain for someone to be guilty: (1) that harm has to have been done – to which he replied, "Doctor, Ethel is dead"; and (2) it has to be the person's responsibility, that there are crimes of commission and crimes of omission, but if someone is careful and a death still occurs, it is sad but accidental and not the person's fault – to which he explained that he blamed himself for her death because while she had consented, it was he who had strongly advocated she have the surgery to restore her capacities for activities that he sought (e.g., sex, travel). I paused, then said, "I don't know if you have any spiritual or religious beliefs, sir, and I don't want to seem presumptuous, but if Ethel were in heaven and could somehow look down, what advice do you think she would give you?" He said, "She'd tell me to snap out of it." I asked, "Why do you think that?" and he replied, "Because she wanted me to be happy – that's why she had the damn operation in the first place." I looked at him and said, "Then wouldn't it be a better way of honoring her memory to everyday do something positive that she would want you to enjoy and say, 'Thank you. I dedicate this to you, dear.'" He looked untroubled as he realized a better way to go forward.

   In another instance, a woman whose partner had also died was being bothered by another woman who had temporarily befriended her but whose attentions were no longer wanted. The client was stuck, feeling unable to get the other woman to desist. As you can see in the videotape I sometimes show at workshops, I said, "Sometimes when I need extra support I think of someone who means a lot to me. What would your friend who died tell you to do?" She smiled. "She'd tell her to butt out – hey, I can do that!"

   In these cases of evoking an internalized other as a resource, I was drawing from both (1) Sigmund Freud (1917) who, in his paper "Mourning and Melancholia," said that we sometimes get stuck in pathological grief because we experience the lost person as a critic or censor (which

I reversed into experiencing the lost person as an ally); and (2) Michael White (1989), the title of whose paper "Saying Hullo Again: The Incorporation of the Lost Relationship in the Resolution of Grief" explains itself. Some of the questions White suggests exploring with grieving clients include:

✓ *If you were seeing yourself through _____'s eyes right now, what would you be noticing about yourself that you could appreciate?*

✓ *What do you know about yourself that you are awakened to when you bring alive the enjoyable things that _____ knew about you?*

✓ *What difference would it make to how you feel if you were appreciating this in yourself right now?*

✓ *In taking this next step, what else do you think you might find out about yourself that could be important for you to know?*

✓ *How could you let others know that you have reclaimed some of the discoveries about yourself that were clearly visible to _____, and that you find personally attractive?*

If someone came in wearing a cross, perhaps we could talk about how Jesus could help them, or if they came in wearing something else and it fit maybe we could talk about what the Holy Quran or the Torah or the Book of Mormon says. I saw a young man with multiple tattoos who was getting into trouble. When I found out that he was into basketball (I'm tall and used to play), I told him about an interview I had read with a popular basketball star who explained the meanings of his "tats," including the one on his arm in honor of his grandmother – and then the young man showed me one on his arm that he carried to inspire himself. The idea is to get them to use their own internal resources – who are their guides, their allies, their strengths, their helpers? I was talking with a woman about a problem she was having with someone, and we were getting nowhere. And then I said, "Who's your favorite superhero?" And she said, "Buffy, Buffy the Vampire Slayer." And I said, "What would Buffy do?" And she said, "She'd kick his ass." And I said, "Well, how would she do that?" And she told me. So I said, "I don't want you to be violent, but could you do something in the spirit of Buffy?" And we laughed, and she said, "Oh, yeah, I can Buffy." And so suddenly, she was calling in one of her allies, one of her resources. In my personal hero pantheon, Buffy the Vampire Slayer is not on the list. But the idea is that people have internal resources that might be useful, whether it's "Mother Mary comes to me" or the Buddha, or maybe Steph Curry or their beloved third-grade teacher or Dr. Milton Erickson or Dr. Martin Luther King. For her, it was Buffy the Vampire Slayer. What are the exceptions to the problem, when isn't the problem a problem and is there somebody who could help them to do that?

Reflection questions: What family member, religious or spiritual figure, mythological character, superhero, historical personage, sports or movie star, celebrity, higher power, etc. could serve as an ally for one (or more!) of your SST clients? How could you invoke them in a session?

_____

_____

_____

_____

_____

_____

_____

_____

- In another instance (reported in Hoyt & Cannistrà, 2023, pp. 46–47), a therapist who was seeing a married couple asked her client "Who's your favorite movie star?" and the man named a charming, debonair fellow. And the therapist said, "Why do you like him?" "Oh, because he's handsome and he's articulate and he's kind and he always gets the girl in the end." And the therapist said, "How would this movie star talk to your wife?" and the man explained how he imagined the star would act and what he would say to her. And the therapist said, "Why don't you pretend you're the movie star and, for the next week, when you begin to have a conflict, act like you're him?" And the guy said, "Well, but…" and the therapist said, "You know, just try it" and the wife laughed and then the therapist reminded him that the star gets the girl in the end. And it worked – he tried it and when he acted nicer the wife responded differently and they got unstuck and things got better. Now, the reason I know about this case is because I was the husband – not the therapist! Otherwise, we could still be writing our check and going every week and talking about male and female roles and communication styles and our childhoods and family-of-origin intergenerational dynamics. Discussing ways to get the most from the session, Dryden (2019b, pp. 213–214) also recommends "Utilize the client's role model" and describes some ways to do so (e.g., identifying the model and similarities between the model and the client, identifying the model's skills and how they operate, educating the client about how to perform the needed skills).

Reflection questions: Who in your life inspires you? How does that happen? How could that be used in a single session?

_____

_____

_____

_____

_____

_____

_____

_____

• Hoyt and Irving Janis (1975) describe a one-session procedure for helping people make and stick to stressful decisions (such as maintaining an exercise program). A motivational balance sheet is developed in which the person lists pros and cons for (a) the emotional and (b) the practical consequences for (c) self and (d) for others of sticking to a certain regimen (e.g., they'll feel happy and lose weight and will be proud of themselves and others will admire their accomplishments versus they'll be unhappy and less healthy and not like themselves and others will be disappointed).

A woman sought therapy wanting to "sort out my thoughts" about whether to continue at a certain job or to seek a different position. In one session, a semi-structured "motivational balance-sheet procedure" was used to help her weigh the implications of her options. Within an hour, she came to her decision, which she recognized as what she had thought she wanted to do. Her choice now felt more "solid," however, and she ended by saying that she had gotten what she had come for, and that she would call again if she needed help in the future (reported in Rosenbaum, Hoyt, & Talmon, 1990/1995, p. 117).

The basic emotional and practical pros-and-cons structure can be adapted to various decisions, such as continuing or not continuing a relationship, staying at a job or in school (or not), moving to a new city or remaining where they are, etc. If the clients have not already made up their minds and are still quite ambivalent, it may be better (*à la* motivational interviewing – see Miller, 2000) to have them voice the positives and have someone else (the therapist, or maybe an imaginary opponent) voice the negatives of a desired course of action.

As a decision-making Socratic variant, the therapist can have a client describe the pros and cons of one option in detail ("Why do you say that?") and then the pros and cons of another option in detail, and then ask the client to imagine that they had been sitting up on the bookcase listening in – "and what would you think and what would you do if you had heard what we've been talking about for the past 20 minutes?"

Reflection questions: What is a single session situation in which you might use a motivational balance sheet procedure? How would you proceed?

• Hoyt (2017, p. 172) describes a situation in which, in one session, a client came to recognize that she would do better if she resumed taking the antidepression medication that she had benefited from previously. In another situation, described in Hoyt (in press), a woman who was benefiting from medication asked to see her psychiatrist for a single session of psychotherapy to discuss a problem. Although the psychiatrist's main professional focus was the use of medications to treat mood disorders, she also appreciated the opportunity to use her psychosocial therapeutic skills. They met for an SST and by focusing on the patient's specific session goals and the skills she could utilize to achieve those goals, the patient got the psychotherapeutic support and direction she had sought; and she continued with her medication regimen.

Reflection question: When might SST be useful within the context of medication?

_____

_____

_____

_____

_____

_____

_____

_____

- In Hoyt (2014/2017, pp. 272–286), I tell the story of "Psychology and My Gallbladder: An Insider's Account of a Single-Session Therapy." Until almost age 60, I had never had any significant medical issues and then had a serious episode of gallbladder illness that was going to require a cholecystectomy. As I detail in the full account, I was very anxious. (Fittingly, I started the published report with an epigraph from the 13th-century Sufi mystic and poet, Rumi, who said "I have lived on the lip of insanity, wanting to know reasons, knocking on the door. It opens. I've been knocking from the inside!") I met with a licensed clinical social worker who used a variety of techniques to help me access resources for better coping and recovery. Some of the features of the SST included:

  ✓ At an initial meeting with some colleague-friends, one of them reassured me and another suggested that I write out and give to the surgeon a list of statements I wanted her to make (and not make) and ask the surgeon to be sure to say them. "That's brilliant," said the other friend, "it puts him in a meta position – you'll still have some control even while you're out." I was also advised to write out an imagery scene I found comforting that we could use when we did our single session.

  ✓ When I met with the therapist in her office, we negotiated a realistic treatment goal (notice her shifting to less anxiety-provoking language, from "pain" to "discomfort" – see Battino, 2010):

    'What do you want to have happen?'
    'I don't want to have any pain, not one iota.'
    'Well, we can't be sure of that. How about: 'I'd like to have the maximum comfort and the least discomfort available in the situation.'
    'Okay.'

✓   The therapist suggested and guided me, "Whatever way would be easiest for you to relax and go into trance. Let me show you what I mean. You may want to write down some notes" and gave me a pen and piece of paper. I have the paper and see what I wrote: "Wise Unconscious – Assist me to do this the wisest way … to use my resources … doing my part …taking care of me. [...]" (See Hammel, 2020, regarding ways to speak that bypass conscious resistance.)

✓   At the hospital, waiting for the surgery, I found myself thinking of my late brother and mother and how they had handled things. I remembered seeing Mom in a challenging situation and heard the words "CALM. COOPERATIVE. COMPETENT. COMFORTABLE" and understood how they could work for me.

✓   Surgery went well. I went home that day, and my recovery was uneventful. When, sometime later, I had to deal with another medical issue, I heard the alliterative CALM, COOPERATIVE, COMPETENT, COMFORTABLE and did fine.

✓   It was a single session with several parts and multiple contributors – friends,[3] surgeon, SST therapist, my wife, late family members – and myself. The therapist helped me connect my resources and goals (see Context of Competence, Chapter 2.) Consistent with Shakespeare's line from *All's Well that Ends Well* (Act I, Scene 1), "Our remedies often in ourselves do lie" (with some help from friends!).

Reflection question: Have you ever had an experience in which, as the result of a single session you personally made a useful shift and/or were able to resolve a problem?[4] What happened?

_____

_____

_____

_____

_____

_____

_____

_____

---

3   With special thanks to Carol Erickson, Murray Korngold, John Frykman – and my Mom.

4   For another example of a professional therapist being an SST client, see Rossi and Rossi (2014).

Do What Works

All of the cases presented here were single sessions. Many SST cases are essentially competency-based strengths-oriented variants of solution-focused therapy (and its postmodern constructivist cousin, narrative therapy – see Chang & Phillips, 1993), Ericksonian hypnosis and strategic therapy, cognitive-behavioral therapy, and even occasionally psychodynamic therapy. Those are approaches I certainly draw upon. I agreed when I saw in Nardone and Portelli's (2005, p. 10) genealogy of brief strategic therapy that they had placed my name in the "Synthetic Models" category that draws from solution-focused therapy (the Milwaukee Model), brief strategic therapy (the Palo Alto Model), and family strategic brief therapy (the Washington Model). Jay Haley (1973, 1985) popularized the term *strategic therapy* (1963) and defined it (1973, p. 1): "Therapy can be called strategic if the clinician initiates what happens during therapy and designs a particular approach for each problem." A related definition was offered by Bob Rosenbaum (1990, p. 354):

> Strategic therapy is not a particular approach or theory [...] It rather refers, in its broadest sense, to any therapy in which the therapist is willing to take on the responsibility for influencing people and takes an active role in planning a strategy for promoting change.

It's good to have options. I recall, for example, one time seeing a family that was not very verbal and thinking "Gee, I should have paid more attention when Virginia Satir (see Constantine, 1978; Satir, 1988; Söderquist, 2023, p. 82) was explaining family sculpting." How about the Internal Family Systems Model (Schwartz, 2023)? Maybe focused Acceptance and Commitment Therapy (Robinson, Strosahl, & Gustavsson, 2012)? One can't know everything, but it's good to know what might be particularly useful in a given situation.

Different techniques may be used to accomplish the same purpose, and different purposes (or "logics" – see Cannistrà, 2019; Cannistrà & Hoyt, 2023) may be served by the same techniques. Barnes, Carruthers, and Gigovic (2018) offer "One…Two…Three Ways to Help You Today" in which they describe how three different therapists – one working from a cognitive-behavioral therapy (CBT) perspective, another from a solution-focused brief therapy (SFBT) perspective, and a third from a narrative therapy perspective – each did a helpful single session with the same client. Of course, if you're going to be *multi-theoretical* (I prefer that term rather than *eclectic*, which sounds like a cross between electric and chaotic, throwing a mixed bag of techniques at the client), the techniques should be mutually compatible and synergistic. I've always liked Scott Miller's (1992) phrase, "symptoms of solution" – seeing emerging little bits of health, not illness. You don't want to squash a solution that is inchoate or *in statu nascendi*. Thus, Robert Neimeyer (1998, pp. 62–63) warns of the "STDs (Serious Theoretical Discrepancies)" that may result from casually commingling therapies infused with contradictory core epistemological values. But, done thoughtfully, as Dryden (2020, p. 283) advised: "[T]he expertise of the therapist when allied to the expertise of the client can be a potent force for good in SST/OAAT therapy."

One size doesn't fit all, and human beings are complex and can be understood in many different ways. Sermijn and Gergen (2017, p. 60) note:

> The traditional practices of asking questions, and careful empathic listening, are severely limited. We are *multi-beings* and if you bring only a single way of being into therapy – the result of training in a specific school of therapy – you are reducing your capacity for effective therapeutic relations.

Cooper and McLeod (2007) and Dryden (2019b, pp. 114–115) also comment favorably on the value of appropriately pluralistic ("both/and" rather than "either/or") practices. If coherent and integrated, techniques can be drawn from an array of theories, but sometimes eclecticism sounds like a version of Luigi Pirandello's (1921/1998) play, *Six Character in Search of an Author*. Gerald Corey (2017, pp. 428–429) warns:

> At its worst, eclectic practice consists of haphazardly picking techniques without any overall theoretical rationale. This is known as *syncretism*, wherein the practitioner, lacking in knowledge and skill in selecting interventions, looks for anything that seems to work, often making little attempt to determine whether the therapeutic procedures are indeed effective. Such an uncritical and unsystematic combination of techniques is no better than a narrow and rigid orthodoxy.

The various approaches and techniques mentioned here are proffered for use, in SST or elsewhere, when they fit. Bill O'Hanlon (1990, pp. 86–87) rightly identified the two tasks of brief therapy as (1) "Changing the viewing," and (2) "Changing the doing." Perhaps the term "mosaic" (see Zeig, 2022b, p. 5) can express the multi-faceted nature of our many human constructions. Again, "The search [is] for a conceptualization that would allow a viable and parsimonious solution. The therapist needs to be versatile, innovative, and pragmatic, asking: 'What would help this [client] today?'" (Hoyt, Rosenbaum, & Talmon, 1992, p. 63). As the preceding examples illustrate, one size (or method) doesn't fit all. *"Do what works"* is a good motto. As Jay Haley (quoted in Crenshaw, 2004, p. 46) said, when asked how he knew to use a certain intervention at a certain time: "You wouldn't use it on someone it wouldn't work on!"

SST in Cross-Cultural Contexts

6

When doing SST, or other therapy, it is important to be cognizant of possible cultural influences. What might make sense in my worldview might not fit so well in someone else's. This can be especially important when attempting to be helpful in one session, since client and clinician need to quickly form an effective working relationship. Recalling the *Context of Competence* discussed in Chapter 2 (see Figure 2.1 on page 29), participants may have different culturally based values and perspectives regarding what constitutes an acceptable Alliance, appropriate Goals, and/or available Resources.

Back in 1995, at an in-house meeting of brief therapists, Jay Haley remarked (quoted in Hoyt, 1997/2000, p. 198):

> Therapy was built upon European immigrants, and now we have the Asian immigrants and the South American immigrants. At a local elementary school near me they had a multicultural day and the kids all came in their costumes. There were 187 cultural groups! And a lot of those are heading for therapy. So, we're going to work with them just hoping they speak English. It's a whole new scheme.

In what follows I first highlight some examples of cross-cultural issues drawn from the SST literature and then describe a few of my own experiences. It is good to know "where the person is coming from" so that you and he/she/they can work together as effectively and efficiently as possible. Unfortunately, we often "discover" cultural differences when there is a clash – which is not likely

DOI: 10.4324/9781003468547-6

to promote successful SST. It is less probable that SST (or other therapy) will be very helpful if the customer is misunderstood, unappreciated, or offended.

The following discussion of SST in cross-cultural contexts is offered to highlight the importance of cultural awareness, humility, and competence.

Some Examples from the SST Literature

We will first consider some cross-cultural observations from the SST literature, giving thumbnail descriptions and highlighting some lessons. Readers are encouraged to consult the original reports for important details.

- John Miller (2014) describes his experience, starting in 2005, of traveling from the U.S. to mainland China to teach and collaborate on research regarding clinical delivery and family therapy. He notes (p. 197) that

  > in the developing Chinese context, family/interpersonally based, short-term, problem-focused, brief, and directive approaches have had the greatest appeal and acceptance among the people. This is likely due to unique aspects of Chinese culture such as 'filial piety' (*xiào*), a Confucian virtue that includes a central value of respect for parents and family ancestors. [...] Generally speaking, Chinese culture values helping professionals who are directive, expert-based, and oriented to solving the problem quickly and pragmatically [...] The single session therapy methods I had been practicing since 1995 seemed to be an ideal fit for the emerging field of therapy in China and the preferences of most people seeking services there.

  He presents several fascinating cases involving family issues. He concludes the chapter by writing (p. 212): "We and the groups we belong to are composed of many interrelated stories and that if we only hear the single story of another individual or group we hazard a critical misunderstanding" and "in China and around the world we can often help clients find their 'better story' in one session."

- Jason Platt and Debora Mondellini (2014) describe their experiences providing walk-in SST for street robbery victims in Mexico City. In a clinical vignette, they illustrate (p. 226) trying to develop a more collaborative stance when developing a therapeutic alliance, saying to the client: "Hmm ... what experience has taught us is that everyone feels, thinks and reacts differently, so it would be impossible for us to be experts on your experience ...maybe we can figure it out together?" They comment (pp. 226–227):

The hierarchical culture in Mexico, as it plays out in therapy, is a constant challenge and a paradox: if we want to proceed with a collaborative approach, are we behaving 'anti-collaboratively' by imposing our beliefs when a client apparently needs or expects us to be more hierarchical? [...] We have found that emphasizing the client's experience and strengths gradually demystifies this notion as the client becomes more empowered.

They note the high incidence of robberies, and the importance of normalizing, not pathologizing, the reactions of victims. They note the cultural reluctance of people to discuss personal problems outside the home, and conclude (p. 230): "We believe that part of our social responsibilities as therapists is to demystify therapy and promote its benefits, and single session therapy – which offers minimalistic constructive intervention as a small, affordable, and accessible safe first step – might just be the ideal way to get us on the way."

• Terry Soo-Hoo (2018), who was born in Hong Kong and moved to the U.S. at age 6, notes (p. 186) that

> many cultural groups view Western psychotherapy (particularly long-term psychotherapy) as something alien to their views of mental-health and illness. [...] Oftentimes people from these cultures enter therapy reluctantly. Even if they come to therapy for help there is the expectation that treatment will be done quickly, perhaps in one session.

He goes on (p. 186):

> the therapist working within an SST model also must work within the client's cultural context or framework. This is especially true due to the time constraints of the model. There really is very little time to cultivate a therapeutic alliance with the client. The therapist must very quickly assess what are the important cultural factors to consider in helping clients find solutions to their presenting problems.

He presents the case of a young Vietnamese-American woman, an oldest daughter, who had seen a previous therapist and been turned off when that therapist recommended that she set a boundary and essentially abandon her troubled father. In contradistinction, in a single session Soo-Hoo helps her to see how she can honor and help her father while *also* taking care of herself. In his discussion, Soo-Hoo comments (p. 199):

In this case, there were a number of key cultural concepts that the therapist needed to consider. One was the understanding that the client viewed family involvements and relationships through the lens of a collectivist culture. The second important point was to listen to the client about what she wanted. [...] Finally, it is important for therapists to pay attention to how clients react to therapeutic interventions. The previous therapist had suggested that she was over-involved with her father and needed to individuate so she could focus more on her own life. Although he was well-intentioned, he ignored the cultural nuances of the situation. [...] This first therapist could have recognized that the intervention was not being received in a positive way and could have reassessed his clinical approach. A culturally competent therapist is able to be flexible and adaptable in finding ways to assist clients that are consistent within their cultural context.

- John Miller, Jason Platt, and Kevin Conroy (2018) describe some of the challenges of service delivery in Cambodia, a country that has been torn by warfare and political strife. They note (pp. 116–117) that

> One of the challenges of our work has been making use of the methods and theories from our Western training in non-Western contexts. While the Western world dominates the field of therapy, it ironically is designed to fit for only a minority of the world's population. The Western world from which most models of psychotherapy emanate represents only about 5% of the global population (Arnett, 2008).

They present accounts of several SSTs, some occurring in harrowing circumstances in countryside villages. They advise (p. 127): 'Humility and trusting in the local expert is the best foundation for presenting single-session interventions. They know the context, cultural values, and how difficulties are conceptualized in Cambodia better than any visiting scholars could possibly know.' They also write (p. 131, italics in original): 'Our work in the majority world has also taught us the importance of maintaining a position of *humility and curiosity* about what is happening' and that

> When encountering the severe and seemingly hopeless situations we have seen in these majority world contexts it can be easy to become overwhelmed and be tempted to give up. [...] Instead we advise others entering this work to *maintain a sense of optimism* about the work. Get involved, and believe that your efforts can and will make a difference.

[…] We encourage therapists engaging in this work to recognize the healing power of simply creating a place or space for people to *tell their stories* and appreciate their sorrows and accomplishments. […] Single-session therapy seems one ideal strategy for better meeting the needs of those living in majority world contexts.

(p. 132)

- Irma Rodriguez (2018) describes how she and colleagues have adapted ideas from Collaborative Therapy (Anderson, 1998; Anderson & Gehart, 2007), single-session therapy (Talmon, 1990), and walk-in services (Slive & Bobele, 2011) at their community-based counseling center in an underdeveloped neighborhood in Mexico City. She notes that they came to call the service *"Terapia breve, sin cita"* ("Brief therapy, no appointment") rather than *"Sesión unica"* ("Single Session Therapy") because the term "single session" was not familiar to the receptionist or to prospective clients – they thought it meant they would only be allowed one visit, rather than the idea of one-session-at-a-time.[1] After describing several interesting cases, she further reflects (p. 301):

I would like to emphasize the difference that the words *unique* and *single* have for me. *Single* invites me to think of each encounter as the only opportunity to meet with a person [this is 'OAAT'] and the responsibility to foster a meaningful conversation that opens possibilities. *Unique* invites me to appreciate, value, and recognize what is unique, special, and different in each person and situation. [This is 'one size doesn't fit all.'] Whether we meet for one session, or more, each encounter brings out the uniqueness of each conversation and relationship. In this process, we have the privilege of becoming the therapist / team that our client needs and that the occasion calls for.

---

1   The 2021 Spanish translation (published by Editorial Eleftheria in Barcelona) of the 2018 Hoyt et al. book title *Single-Session Therapy by Walk-In or Appointment* is *Terapia de una Sola Sesión con o sin Cita Previa*. Martin Söderquist (2023, p. 44) in Sweden reports: "The concept SST can be misleading. On one occasion a man called me and wanted to schedule a single session and I asked as I usually do: 'Who will join you?' and the guy briefly said: 'I will come alone – it is single session.' We did find out the slight misunderstanding (but of course he could come to session alone) and scheduled the session. Later we changed from single session to OAAT." For further discussion of the ways the term *single session therapy* has been rendered in other languages, see examples below and Hoyt et al. (2021, pp. 14–15).

- John Miller, Dai Xing, Hu Yaorui, and Xu Yilin (2021) describe the development of a single session therapy service in China. They note (p. 245) that at the beginning of their work,

    there was not an immediately translatable word for the concept of 'therapy' in the Chinese language at the time. Over the past few years the Chinese therapy community has adopted the Chinese [Mandarin] term for 'family treatment' (*Jiāting liáofǎ*) to express the concept of family therapy. The term we have adopted to reflect the one-time nature of the meeting is 'single session and brief' (*Dān jié jiânjiè*).

    Using feedback from Chinese colleagues and clients, a seven-step Single Session Team Family Therapy (SSTFT) protocol was created, with each Chinese client family being seen over a three-hour period. Each of the therapists takes turns bringing a family for the SSTFT, with the other therapists serving as an observing/reflecting team and the lead author supervising. In their conclusion (p. 252), Miller et al. note

    We have found that one advantage of this method lies in the ability of the team to capitalize on the 'wisdom of the crowd,' [...] that the group as a whole is often wiser than any one individual in the group. This idea is very consistent with Chinese culture's focus on communal collaboration and collectivism as an ancient core value. In our experience, this method of team consultation matches the Chinese tendency to 'gather around' a problem in an effort to solve it as a group.

    They also note (pp. 252–253) the rich two-way exchange of ideas between Eastern and Western therapists, and that

    Given that the majority of the world's population lives within about a 3000-mile radius of Shanghai, there is much to learn about how these 'majority world' families live and work (Miller, Platt, & Conroy, 2018). As Confucius tells us ['The man who moves a mountain begins by carrying away small stones'], big changes often originate from small actions. This is consistent with our understanding of the practice of single session therapy throughout the world.

- Alison Elliott, James Dokona, and Henry von Doussa (2021) present, using a conversational format consistent with the oral traditions of Indigenous cultural work, a discussion about using single session approaches with Aboriginal families in the state of Victoria, Australia. They describe the importance of listening carefully and respectfully to people who have been marginalized/colonized – rather than the counselor setting the goal and the pace of the meeting. The counselor may announce the time frame ("one hour") but the content, how to use the time, is up to the family. For example, in one passage (p. 214, emphasis in original) James says:

> When I meet with the family I see the conversation is like a river running: you never know which way it's going to go. The challenge with some other frameworks is the idea of interviewing the family to develop a hypothesis as to what's happening. And I feel *that in doing this, already the balance of power has gone towards the worker/therapist.* The SST model doesn't do that. You go in and you see the family where they are and explore how they've been managing and what they want to get out of the conversation.

He describes letting the family know that an hour has been reserved for the meeting and then allowing the clients to decide how to use the time. A few exchanges later (p. 215), Alison elaborates:

> I did want to talk about listening and taking in information because to me it talks to *Dadirri*[2] – that sense of, if you listen deeply without coming up with something as the worker or the therapist, that gives agency straight away to the client because it's giving space for a possible different way of thinking. If you've always been disempowered, where someone's been telling you what to do next (which is colonization in its essence), then it feels like somebody's thought that they know better than you. Listening deeply helps us to pause and really get to what's most important right now and allows nature's timing. Life's the teacher, we're not going to be in their life all the time, that kind of thing is good to keep in mind too. *Dadirri* fits well within a single session framework as the very concept and way of being is to trust, wait for the right time for things and to develop a deeper awareness of when to act and when not to, when to speak and when to be silent. And to be comfortable with not knowing the answers.

---

2   A footnote in the original chapter (Elliott et al., 2021, p. 222) explains: "*Dadirri* is a word that belongs to the language of the Ngangikurrungur peoples of Daly River in the Northern Territory. The activity or practice of *Dadirri* is a way of cultivating a deep level of mind awareness, listening to self and others. It has its equivalent word and meaning in many other Indigenous groups across the continent of Australia."

- Sophia Sorensen (2021) describes her experience of providing Single Session Therapy in Indigenous (First Nation) communities in Canada. She observes protocols that involve services never being presumptive but rather always requested by the leadership of a specific Indigenous community, counseling services always being delivered on traditional lands, her first task once in community being to connect with village leadership, and that the group would determine action items, location, time, and possible inclusion of other healers. Drawing from her training in Collaborative Therapy at the Houston Galveston Institute (see Levin, Gil-Wilkerson, & Rapini De Yatim, 2018) as well as other experiences, she recounts meeting with a man who appeared to be in his late 40s. After first hearing about various traumas and difficulties, and the man asking the unanswerable question *"Why?"* all these terrible things had happened, they moved to consider *"How?"* – such as how he survived, how he made decisions that helped him to cope, how he knew when to ask for help. She notes that the SST approach is extremely well-suited for working with Indigenous clients for many reasons, including that the walk-in format removes a barrier and allows for spontaneity, the client's anticipation of only one session translates into a sense of freedom, plus meeting outside of an office setting and allowing the client to determine the session length increases client comfort and trust. She also writes (p. 231, emphasis in original):

    Finally, and perhaps most importantly, Indigenous clients often have experienced long periods of a lack of respect and lack of positive endorsement. For this reason, approaching this client group with the mindset that *clients are the experts in their own lives* is especially empowering and sometimes a rare, almost radically empowering experience.

- Bronwyn Dunnachie, Stacey Porter, and Karin Isherwood (2021) provide an account of their efforts to implement Single Session Family Consultation (SSFC; see O'Hanlon & Rottem, 2021, discussed in Chapter 4) in *Aotearoa* New Zealand. Māori and Pasifika peoples (and others) had attended a conference presentation led by staff from The Bouverie Centre (based in Melbourne, Australia), as well as SSFC workshops in Auckland and Wellington, and gave feedback that the SSFC framework (p. 236) "could work well in the *Aotearoa* New Zealand context, although the resources and language would require cultural consideration and a specific consultation plan." After further meetings with a Māori cultural advisor and providers, it was determined that successfully convening an

SSFC with Māori *whanau* [family] may include protocol additions such as these (p. 241):

✓   Understanding the service users' and their *whanau*'s traditional needs
✓   Accommodating speaking in their own language
✓   Expecting to include *tamariki* [children] and *mokopuna* [grandchildren]
✓   Providing appropriate *manaakitanga* [hospitality, such as food and drink].[3]

As Dunnachie et al. note (p. 242), recommendations "highlighted the need for services to seek local support and cultural advice, set quality improvement expectations in policy and procedure, and support self-reflective practice with emphasis on understanding one's own cultural practice before engaging safely with another's."

•   Brian Guthrie (2018) reflects on his experience of providing SST in Haiti two years after the major disaster of the January 2010 earthquake. He notes (p. 305) that

Culturally, in Haiti mental-health problems are often attributed to supernatural forces, with problems in daily functioning often viewed as the consequence of a spell, a hex, or a curse cast by a jealous person. Mental illness is also attributed to the failure to please spirits, including those of deceased family members.

In his account, he recalls the moment (p. 307, emphasis in original) when "I sat with my first client in the open air shaded by the wall of the clinic. For the first time as a therapist, I was confronted with the stark reality of *one session is all I have*." He goes on to write (p. 307):

Often the intervention was simply offering advice to the client, reframing the problem, or normalizing what the patient perceived as abnormal or unusual. In almost every situation the acknowledgment and

---

3   This reminds me of what writer-photographer Will Baker (1983, p. 262) said about his two attempted encounters with conventional psychiatry during times of despair: "Both times, and only those times, I had gone to see the shaman of my own culture, the psychiatrist, I learned, this past night [spent around the fire with Indian friends], what had been missing from those sessions – which I very soon abandoned – missing from those offices with their polished wood, filing cabinets, soft lighting and black leather. There was nothing to drink. There was no singing. There was no ring of honest old friends with a yen to talk. There were no small boys to occupy the lap, or to tickle the feet."

validation of the tremendous grief and loss of loved ones provided a cathartic experience.

Guthrie explains that he used reframing to enable clients to view the problem as more manageable and to then help them identify existing resources that they could use to resolve the reframed view of their presenting problem. He presents a case in which he helps a bereft woman, first commending her for the love she had for her children and the importance of keeping their memories alive, and then focusing on her beginning to experience how she might remember her children. He asks her to tell him about the children and what she loved about each, what they would want her to do, and which memories they would hope she would keep close to her heart. He also, in closing the session, taught her some practical stress management techniques to address her initial problem of insomnia and anxiety. He notes (p. 309) that "I followed the three primary assessment questions of SST: (1) How is the client stuck?; (2) What does the client need to get unstuck?; and (3) How can I provide or facilitate what is needed? (Hoyt, 1990, 1994)." He also remarks on the importance of therapist self-care when working in such extraordinarily dire circumstances. For some other accounts of using SST principles in humanitarian crisis situations, see Nùñez and Abia (2021, summarized below), Miller (2011), Akerele and Yuryev (2017), van der Veer (2017), Bisson (2003), and Paul and van Ommeren (2013).

• Rafael Nùñuz and Jorge Abia (2021) describe using single session Ericksonian strategic hypnotherapy in Mexico to aid disaster survivors (p. 256):

> We see single session hypnotherapy occupying a particular niche within an array of more traditional therapeutic services. Our work deals with developing and testing specific techniques for clear-cut goals. Sometimes one session is all that is possible – and all that is needed.

They provide accounts of single session interventions in village public squares with groups of 20–200 people a few days after terrible earthquakes struck in September 2017. Whole villages participated together. After explaining the procedures and gaining participants' consent, group inductions were conducted. As the authors write (p. 260):

> In strategic Ericksonian hypnotherapy, the use of metaphors facilitates the understanding of the problem and the elaboration of solutions. [...] Metaphors are designed that are specific for each group or

community. Thanks to this […] we were able to adapt and intervene in Indigenous communities that do not speak Spanish.

They describe and give examples of group hypnotherapy inductions and present before-and-after data as evidence of single session effectiveness.

- In our 2023 book, *Brief Therapy Conversations: Exploring Efficient Intervention in Psychotherapy* (Hoyt & Cannistrà, 2023, pp. 9–10), Flavio and I had this exchange:

MICHAEL: You were just in London and you were at the BRIEF training and it was with mostly English people, British people. And you're an Italian. Do you have any ideas about how is it different to make an alliance in English with British people instead of in Italy with Italians? If I was going to come to Italy and try to do therapy and I said,

Flavio, what should I know to make a quick alliance with an Italian? Tell me – is there something I should say? Is there a certain way I should act? Do I look them in the eye? Do I shake hands? What's different between Italians and English? Of course, these are obviously big stereotypes

FLAVIO: Very good question. Like Erickson said: 'Observe, observe, observe.' With English people, you need to give many more verbal feedbacks: 'Oh, good. Yeah, that's fine.' In Italy, in my experience, it's usual for me to be more moderate and to give fewer verbal feedbacks while the person is talking. And another thing in England is to be more careful about the distance, you know, the physical distance but also the psychological, emotional distance, even a verbal distance. The sentence, 'Oh, this is very personal!' seems more common there in England than in Italy. I mean, here (in Italy) it's not so common when considering a problem to ask for the person to disclose something 'personal' – we just do that, that's all. It seems to me that the idea to be politically correct is more felt from British and Americans, too. In Italy, you don't need to pay attention to every single word you say because of the racial or sexual implications. Sometimes it's really bad, because there's a lack of awareness about how words work and also about important topics – for example, women's roles. Sometimes it could be good, because there's a more relaxed climate. Italians tend to think that you said something in good faith and don't blame you. If you say, 'Sorry, I didn't know' they will usually reply, 'Don't worry. It's okay.'

MICHAEL: OK. More active feedback with the English and more asking permission to talk about personal things. You have to be more: 'Yeah, yeah. That's interesting.'

These are broad generalities, of course, but illustrate that although the dissimilarities may be greater when Westerners work with people from Asia, Latin America, a Caribbean island, or Indigenous cultures, therapists may still need to adjust somewhat when working with people of various nationalities, cultures, and social groups from the same region or continent.

Some Cross-Cultural Examples from My Own SST Practice

Allow me to situate myself. I am a white, tall, cisgender heterosexual American male, now (2023) in my mid-70s, well educated, upper middle class, married. My wife and I have one adult son who moved away to attend college and then lived on his own for some time; he is now married and lives with his wife in another city. I am secular Jewish and my political views are generally liberal. I mention these factors because they all influence how I see the world, and how the world may see me.

At the risk of stereotyping, here are some stories of my adventures bumping into culture when attempting to do (or teach) Single Session Therapy. Other than the Japanese example, they occurred at an HMO clinic which serves a large and ethnically diverse population. With each case, after describing my well-intended but awkward responses, I will attempt to offer some reflections on lessons learned.

- A Filipino-American woman sought help regarding what she felt was a loss of closeness and affection in her marriage. Learning on the telephone that her husband spent a lot of time with his family, I expected that we might just need a single conjoint session. When she and her husband came in, based on my (mis)reading of structural family therapy (Minuchin, 1974), I quickly suggested that the man should spend less time with his family of origin and more time with his family of election. They looked at me as though I were from another planet (I was!).

Therapy went nowhere, but they were polite and decided to make another appointment with me.

I knew I had missed something, so I consulted with a Filipino-American psychologist-colleague. When I told him what I had said, he shook his head incredulously:

"You really asked him not to see his Mom or go over to help his brothers on the weekend?"

"Well, yeah, kind of – what should I do?"

My consultant was gentle: "Did you ever ask the lady what would make her feel more cared about, or what used to happen that she liked that has stopped happening?"

"Ahhh, no ..."

At the next session, I apologized for my premature suggestion, commented that I needed some more information, and then asked the wife what the husband used to do that she missed: "Oh, he would leave a little love note on the windshield of my car, or call and leave a sweet message on my voicemail at work." (No mention of dumping Mom or the brothers!) I looked over at the husband. He smiled, so I encouraged him to do more of what the wife liked and advised that she let him know how much she liked it. They came back, reported that things were getting better between them, and told me how helpful therapy was.

Lesson: Don't assume you know what's best – ask the clients what has worked and what would work for them.

• The two women made an appointment to see me after hearing that I had a special interest in couple therapy (see Hoyt, 2015). They were both professionals, smart and well dressed, and wanted to discuss some communication issues they were having. After we talked for a few minutes, I (somewhat coyly) asked:

"You're Black and gay and I'm white and straight. Do you think that will be a problem?"

One of the women looked directly at me and said: "For whom?"

Lesson: Don't put it on the clients. Possible cross-cultural issues involve both client(s) and therapist: it's not THEM (unilateral), it's US (bi-personal).

• I recall a time in Japan in which I presented the case of the Woman with the Intrusive Father (Hoyt & Talmon, 1990; Hoyt, 2000/2017) that was discussed in Chapter 4 (see pp. 119–120). I showed a videotape clip from the single session in which I strongly encouraged the young woman to set a boundary and tell her highly intrusive father to "go away" and literally shut the door in his face. It may have been helpful in the U.S., but the Japanese audience informed me that "It would not be possible here to say that to a parent." (When we discussed in what situation such an intervention might be acceptable, I was told: "maybe with a very rude coworker.") In another instance, also in Japan, I requested feedback from an audience, asking what had and had not been helpful. My translator whispered to me, "They can't answer that question the way you asked it – they won't criticize the *sensei* [esteemed teacher]."

> *Lessons:* It would have been better to have asked the audience how one might set a boundary or otherwise deal with an inappropriate parent, rather than assuming that what might be difficult but acceptable in the U.S. would also be acceptable in Japan. (I had proceeded ignorant of the vital role of family obligations.) It would also have been better had I been more aware of how to elicit feedback about the workshop.

Another time in Japan I presented my paper, "A Golfer's Guide to Brief Therapy (with Footnotes for Baseball Fans)" (Hoyt, 1996a/2017). My Japanese discussant scolded me: "You are in Japan and you should use Japanese examples, not ones from golf and baseball." He was perhaps right, although his tone was harsh – and some Japanese do play golf and they have a long tradition of baseball, including Babe Ruth playing there in 1934. (And recently, Shohei Otani is an All-Star in the U.S. as both a pitcher and a hitter.) My discussant's instruction stayed with me. When I spoke at a subsequent conference in Osaka, I started with a bow and modest apology for possibly boring the audience, called the other presenters *sensei*, and quoted Ichiro Suzuki, the great Japanese player now enshrined in the Baseball Hall of Fame in Cooperstown, New York (see Hoyt, 2019a). I also recited three SST haiku (!) that I had written (Hoyt, 1996b, p. 375), the third of which alludes to the legend of the three Japanese lords of old at the local castle in Osaka who revealed their very different characters when asked what they would do with a nightingale that did not sing:

Solution focus
Find exception and increase
Otherwise stay same

More of same, no change
More of difference, not same
When will you notice?

Single session now
Kill it, make it sing, or wait
The cage is open

* Once in my office in Northern California (as recounted in Hoyt, 2017, pp. 221–222), I instructed a young boy from a Mexican American family to "look your father right in the eye and promise him that you'll do better." The boy squirmed a bit, and the session ended inconclusively. When I called to see what happened, the mother explained that the boy had become frightened when I told him to stare at his father's eyes, and "I am sorry, Doctor, but now Octavio is saying that he has a stomachache and doesn't want to come back."

> *Lessons.* The idea of having the boy show respect toward the father was good, but as I learned, in Octavio's world a respectful child doesn't "look your father right in the eye" – and worse, he was in a terrible double-bind, because if he didn't do what *El Doctor* said, then he was disrespecting the doctor! So, what did he do? Well, when you can't win, you don't want to play: a stomachache got him off the hook. Later, teaching in Mexico, in another circumstance involving a family, I had learned enough cultural humility to ask, "How can you show respect for your father?" rather than from my American perspective telling the boy and family what to do.

* The gentleman and his wife appeared to be in their mid-60s. They were dressed formally and she was wearing a hijab head covering. They had sought an appointment "to discuss a problem with the family." They seemed like pleasant, nice people but he very much dominated the discussion and often spoke for her. When I got tired of his near-monologue (I thought "Boy, would my wife be annoyed") and interrupted him and

said, "Let's hear what your wife thinks," *she* responded: "I want to hear what my husband says." He went on, she smiled beatifically, and at the end of the single session, they both said the meeting had been very helpful and thanked me.

Lessons. Some of this pattern may have been due to personality styles, but as I learned from consulting with colleagues who knew the community, it was also consistent with husband/wife role expectations (at least in public, with a stranger) for conservative people of their ethnicity and generation. I had not asked specifically how they wanted me to be helpful, and they had not asked me to address how they communicated with one another. They had sought an appointment to discuss a family problem and seemed happy with the way the session went.

Further Reflections

Hoyt, Young, and Rycroft (2021, p. 337) observed:

> Interestingly, we learn that Australian Aboriginal clients find it healing to know how long a session may last but find it NOT helpful to be directed regarding content, and that *Aotearoa* New Zealand Māori may be offended by being told that they are restricted to a specific time frame; but that Chinese clients seen by Miller et al. want structure and direction by experts! Coming from their different backgrounds, histories, and beliefs, different cultures want different approaches and SST can accommodate them all – but in different ways.

When considering the possibility of SST, it is good to remember that culture may influence how people (including clients and clinicians) form alliances and conceive goals. Culture may also influence the pace at which we expect change to occur. Different groups also may have a tendency to place more emphasis on the past, the present, or the future. Do they want to look backward and review what has happened, talk about the present situation, or mostly let the past go and look forward? Michael Yapko (1989, 1990b) noted that three factors determine whether a client will benefit from brief (including SST) interventions: (1) the person's primary temporal orientation (toward past, present, or future); (2) the general value given to "change," whether he or she is more invested in maintaining tradition or seeking change; and (3) the client's belief system about what constitutes a complete therapeutic experience. Different cultures may structure time differently.

In addition to cultural differences based on nationality, ethnicity, race, language, and religion, we often see the Other through the lenses of politics, social class, educational level, intelligence, geographic origins, physical types, disabilities, style of dress, accents and speech patterns, gender, age differences, degree of psychological mindedness, etc.

These are big generalities, of course.

Culture may influence whether people want the therapist to exercise more (or less) authority, may want more (or less) instruction or advice, may want the therapist to be more (or less) formal. In one context, clients asking the therapist personal questions such as "Are you married? Do you have children? Where did you go to school? Do you go to church?" and perhaps even offering a small gift may seem intrusive; in another context, however, this may be part of the clients building trust. When I Googled *personalismo*, I read: "The concept of *personalismo*, often defined as 'formal friendliness,' basically means that Latinos place great emphasis on personal relationships. Latin culture is both people-oriented and collectivist, meaning that Latinos generally value personal relationships over status, material gain, and institutional relationships" (Foster, 2009).

Perhaps obvious, but worth remembering: "Latinos" (or "Americans," or "New Yorkers," or "Christians," etc.) are not a monolithic group. As Anthony Bourdain (2007, p. 290) remarked in *Kitchen Confidential*:

> Also, learn as much as you can about the distinct cultures, histories and geographies of Mexico, El Salvador, Ecuador and the Dominican Republic. A cook from Puebla is different in background from a cook from Mexico City. Someone who fled El Salvador to get away from the Mano Blanco is not likely to get along with the right-wing Cuban working next to him. [...] Show them some respect by bothering to know them. Learn their language. Eat their food. It will be personally rewarding and professionally invaluable.

The idea that therapy should be an on-going series of 50-minute sessions is a cultural construct. As Flavio Cannistrà and I (Hoyt & Cannistrà, 2023, p. 62) also said in *Brief Therapy Conversations*:

FLAVIO: And this reminds me about Jay Haley (1990), who said that you need to be taught to do a long-term therapy – otherwise it is natural to do brief therapies.

MICHAEL: Five hundred years ago, if I had a problem, I would go and talk to the shaman or the medicine man or woman or the guru or the chief or the village wise person. I would not expect that I'm going to go Tuesday at 10:00 a.m. for 50 minutes once a week for the next two years. I would go to have a meeting and it might not be 50 minutes, it might be all day [a single session!]. I may have to prepare myself to receive the message. [...] And at the end of the experience, I would have ideas and things I'm supposed to do. It's not necessarily that everything is all instantly better, but we developed a very different way of thinking about therapy. I recall Haley (1990, pp. 14–15) saying that the most important decision in the history of therapy was to charge by the hour. People come every week, week after week. They are taught to expect to go gradually and slowly. For some problems, it does take a long time. I'm not against therapy taking as long as it needs. I'm against therapy taking longer than it needs to take and I'm against telling people it has to be a long time.[4]

Considering the way different cultures may employ different means toward the same goals, I also recall Steve de Shazer, who was American, describing something he had observed through his relationship with his wife, Insoo Kim Berg, who was Korean (from Hoyt, 2001, p. 165):

She was raised in a different culture, and I've been studying that culture for 20 years or whatever it is now. There are big differences between Asian and American families. Both of them in general produce reasonable, functional adults. The difference between the two can be sketched this way. In the United States, if a kid does something wrong, he is likely to be grounded. That is, he is imprisoned within the family. Therefore, being with the family is negative – it's a punishment. In Asia, this same kid for the same offense is likely to be expelled from the family in some way. So being with the family is a positive. And we wonder why our families are disintegrating. Why kids can't wait to get

---

4 The etiologies and remedies that we consider are also constructs. As James Hillman and Michael Ventura (1992, p. 17) commented: "If you're out of your mind in another culture or quite disturbed or impotent or anorexic, you look at what you've been eating, who's been casting spells on you, what taboo you've crossed, what you haven't done right, when you last missed reference to the gods or didn't take part in the dance, broke some tribal custom. Whatever. It could be thousands of other things – the plants, the water, the curses, the demons, the gods, being out of touch with the great spirit. It would never, never be what happened to you with your mother and your father 40 years ago. Only our culture uses that model, that myth."

away. The Koreans wonder how they will ever get rid of their kids. It does seem to be exactly the opposite. They both work in the long run; they produce reasonable adults.

"Speak the client's language" doesn't necessarily refer to being fluent in Spanish or Japanese or Hindi or Arabic or Chinese or English, of course, but more generally means being attuned to the client's values and intentions, to the message, the metaphors and terminology, the formality or informality of their speech and nonverbal communication. We should listen and speak in ways that accurately convey both information and respect, varying our style enough to connect with different folks. "Speak the client's language" doesn't just refer to world languages, of course. There are also vernacular nuances ("How's that sound, y'all?"). One time, I started to ask a very unfanciful Silicon Valley engineering guy, "Suppose a miracle happens ..." and he interrupted me: "Doctor, I don't believe in miracles and I don't believe in Santa Claus or the Easter Bunny either." And I said, "Of course. Okay, well, suppose we proceed in a stepwise fashion and you make incremental changes, and the progressive trajectory is consistent with your targeted intention." And he said, "Oh, in that case ..." and laid out what his next steps would be. Speaking the client's language helps to build rapport more quickly. To be effective in SST, the therapist should be, as Arnold Lazarus (1993) nicely put it, an "authentic chameleon."

Kenneth Gergen (1993, p. xi) has written:

> With the mushrooming of communication technologies the stage was set for a vast proliferation of voices. We are saturated by a profusion of opinions, factual claims, theories, critiques, and hypotheses – often conflicting – from around the globe. In effect, we inhabit increasingly a multivocal world, and living viably in this world virtually demands a form of mutilingualism – an ability to shuttle among the domains of intelligibility, to see, and reflexively to see, the peculiarities of one's seeing.

Matt Englar-Carlson (2024, p. xi) concurs:

> Existing and emerging theories of psychotherapy are also challenged to expand beyond the primarily Western worldview endemic in most psychotherapy theories and the practice of psychotherapy itself. That revision and correction requires theories and psychotherapists to become inclusive of the full range of human diversity to reflect an

understanding of human behavior that accounts for a client's context, identity, and intersectionality.

(American Psychological Association, 2017)

We need to learn both *about* and *from* one another. Approached appropriately, many clients from different cultures will find benefit in SST. Getting to know folks from other backgrounds, using cultural consultants, traveling, and reading (e.g., Boyd-Franklin, 2003; McGoldrick, Giordano, & Garcia-Preto, 2005; Sue & Sue, 2013; Hardy & Bobes, 2016) are all helpful. Honesty, curiosity, and respect can go a long way – and we have a long way to go.

What Can We Learn from Our Internalized Clients?[1]

7

Most of us have sometime had the experience of a successful one-session therapy – we met once, something good came of it, and there were no other meetings. As mentioned in the Preface, one of the learning objectives of this book, in addition to introducing ideas about single session/one-at-a-time thinking and practice, is to help readers better identify (and then, it may be hoped, more likely repeat) what they did when they were efficient and effective providers of SST (see Steenbarger, 2012, p. 123).

In what follows, an *internalized other questioning* exercise is presented in which we can learn more about what we did that was helpful in a successful SST.[2] The exercise was originally developed with my colleague, David Nylund (Hoyt & Nylund, 1997/2000). Instructions and guideline questions follow. It takes a bit to get into it, but then interesting discoveries and greater appreciations often occur. One participant described the experience as "like

---

1 Part of the material in this chapter is from "The Joy of Narrative: An Exercise for Learning from Our Internalized Clients," by M.F. Hoyt & D. Nylund, *Journal of Systemic Therapies*, 1997, 16(4), 361–366. ©Guilford Press, 1997. Used with permission.

2 There are also other exercises, of course, that can help us to become more aware of the potential power of an SST. Rycroft and Young (2014) and Cannistrà and Piccirilli (2021), for example, describe several training processes they use to facilitate reflection about mindset and ways to co-create with the client a shared session goal, access resources, ways to stay on track, and how to end successfully.

DOI: 10.4324/9781003468547-7

an oxygen tank"; another likened it to "an autologous transfusion." (That's when some of your own blood is set aside and then given back to you in surgery.) In workshops, I suggest that folks form small groups to do the exercise, since some learn more as the subject, some as the interviewer, and some as an observer – and that way, everyone doesn't have to be on the spot and be a good actor. If done in a small group, once you've done the exercise, you may want to switch and do it again – with different people taking the various roles – and then share what you may have learned. The exercise can also be done by just one person (you!), who reads and answers the different questions.

Internalized other questioning (see Tomm, 1992; Tomm, Hoyt, & Madigan, 1998; McNeel, 1976; Goulding & Goulding, 1979; Nylund & Corsiglia, 1993; Pare, 2008; Vasconcelos & Neto, 2004) offers the opportunity to experience the process of reflexivity, the construction of self via the internalization of significant others.[3] The purpose of the exercise is to help us "re-member" (White, 1997) our skills, abilities, and intentions, to help therapists use our empathy and connectedness as a source of instruction and renewal. It is based on assumptions of curiosity rather than certainty, redolent of "possibilities" and evocative of vocabularies of "solution" rather than "problem."

Be sure to attend to the questions "How will you remember and recall what you have been learning here? When you feel tired or frustrated, what about this client's experience will help encourage you? When you need it, how will you remember to remember?" In my office, there are various little knick-knacks on the shelves. They probably seem inconsequential to most people, but to me they serve as reminders of hope and joy – the grateful teenage girl who gave me the heart-shaped LOVE button, the elderly man who brought me back a souvenir from his trip abroad, the rose (now dried) from the lady who, after our session went outside and picked it and then knocked on my door. What might you learn by recalling SST clients?

---

3   The idea that we form our sense of self by incorporating the views of others is not new. The Roman poet Virgil around 30 BCE said "the many in the one" (*E pluribus unum*); the sociologist Charles Cooley (1902) spoke of the "looking-glass self"; George Herbert Mead (1934) developed symbolic interactionism in *Mind, Self, and Society;* in 1975 Bob Dylan sang "If You See Her, Say Hello" and told us that a part of his girlfriend still lived inside of him and that they had never been apart.

Surprised by Joy, or Were You Expecting Her/Him?[4] What Can We Learn from Our Internalized Clients?

Introduction: The practice of *internalized other questioning* refers to the idea that the "self" is made up of a person's internalized community of significant others. One can "step into" the experience of the other by being addressed by the name of the other person and being asked a series of questions. What can our internalized clients offer to nurture and sustain us?

Invitation: Break into small groups. Now, think of a specific person (client) you have worked with in SST or other brief therapy that had a significant impact on you and your work as a therapist. Imagine that person as best you can – the way they talked, what they said, their intonation, how they sat, how they looked, and so forth. Immerse yourself in the experience. Now, using the practice of internalized other questioning, have your partner interview you *as your client*. The interviewer should function like a reporter or journalist, simply trying to get "the story." He or she should attempt to draw out specific details and particulars (who, what, where, when, how) to increase verisimilitude but should not attempt to "therapize" (change or modify) the client-therapist interviewee. Just try to find out what happened that made the SST a success.

The following are some questions that you may use as guideposts (feel free to devise and ask your own questions). Interview from the internalized other position for about 10–15 minutes.

- What impact did your therapist, _____, have on you? What did you value most about her or him, as a therapist and as a person?
- What would you want your therapist to know about your work together? Were there some things you wish you would have said to her/him? What else? What kept you from sharing this with your therapist?
- What did your therapist do that helped your sense of hope and optimism? What else?
- What submerged strengths and energy did your therapist touch? What did she or he miss?
- Was there a "critical moment" or situation that especially captures or symbolizes how your therapist worked with you in helpful ways? What was said? What happened?

---

4 A nod to C.S. Lewis (1956) for the book title: *Surprised by Joy*. The recent (2024) movie, *Freud's Last Session*, depicts a powerful one-session encounter between Freud and Lewis.

- If you were to tell your therapist something she/he may not have known (or not fully appreciated) about her/his effect on you, what would that be? What would you say?
- Did your therapist share what positive effects your work had on her/him? If so, what was that like? If not, how would you have experienced that?

Now, step out of your client's experience and return to being interviewed as yourself (10–15 minutes). Have somebody ask these questions (or invent your own):

- When you get in touch with your client's experience, what counseling abilities do you most appreciate about yourself?
- What effect will it have on your work knowing how much you impacted your client's life?
- How does getting in touch with these abilities and effects fit with why you became a therapist?
- What colleagues/friends/previous supervisors/clients support these intentions? How? Who would be glad, even honored, to know of your work with the client? What would they say – what words might they use?
- What did your client stimulate in you that you want to nurture and expand? Where is your sense of humor in your clinical work? Your spirit of adventure?
- Do clients get inspired by your sense of hope and passion? How?
- What about your client's experience invigorates you? What gives you joy?
- How will you remember and recall what you have been learning here? When you feel tired or frustrated, what about this client's experience will help encourage you? When you need it, how will you remember to remember?

Now switch roles: The interviewer becomes the interviewee and vice versa. Again, work through the internalized other questions for 10–15 minutes; then interview as self for 10–15 minutes.

Before Closing: The exercise invites a greater awareness of one's influence and the need for accountability and clarity about personal ethics. It is not intended to be a solipsistic stroll through a hermetically sealed hall of mirrors, nor is it intended to indulge clinical incompetence or self-congratulatory arrogant grandiosity. Discussing the experience of the exercise with colleagues is very important, lest one become isolated without recourse to extra-self input. Questions to consider might include:

- Why was this client chosen to reflect upon?
- How do we know the client's wishes and autonomy were honored?
- What ideas might the interviewer and/or other colleagues contribute to help further the therapeutic endeavor?

Summary, Additional Considerations, and Next Steps

8

Single session thinking and practice offers exciting and rewarding possibilities. SST is optimistic and respectful. The therapist needs to be versatile, innovative, and pragmatic, drawing on clients' hopes and resources and focusing on helping them to achieve their goals. When I consider the merits of a (brief) therapy approach, I look at three things: (1) *effectiveness and efficiency:* Does it work, or more nuanced, with whom (and how) is it likely to work? (2) *ethics:* Does it respect and enhance the client's sense of self-autonomy? and (3) *aesthetics:* Is it interesting and attractive, does it capture the listener's ear? The various SST methods we have described are intended to fit the bill on all three counts.

The research and extensive clinical experience are clear, and more and more therapists, managers, and policymakers are embracing SST. For some, though, it may be that a limiting mindset (a hidebound ideology or underlying theory or belief, perhaps along with financial incentives) makes it hard to accept the evidence that for many, one session of psychotherapy can help and may all that is wanted or needed. When I read one colleague's rearguard and inaccurate statement that "SST is not therapy, it's coaching," I thought "It's okay to have your own opinion, but not your own facts." I recalled something two of my colleagues (Slive & Bobele, 2019a, p. 16) wrote: "In an era of a well-intentioned focus on evidence-based practices, it is ironic that the evidence that supports SST is unknown to or ignored by many professionals." I also thought of the work that two other colleagues (Young & Jebreen, 2020) did to debunk a misguided effort by critics to deny licensure credits by falsely claiming that SST was not therapy. I appreciated the four

DOI: 10.4324/9781003468547-8

international SST symposia, the numerous books, the dozens of research studies, and the many thousands of clinical hours from all over the world that have demonstrated that while SST is not a panacea that solves everything, a single session of therapy is often all that someone requires to help them with a variety of mental health issues. (You can Google "Single Session Therapy" and see the most recent information for yourself.) Single session thinking and practice are expanding and going global.

SST in a Nutshell Redux

All the cases presented herein have in common that they were single sessions. The basics of SST are working in a collaborative and culturally appropriate way:

1. Plan for one visit ("one-at-a-time")
2. Identify the client's goal for the session (which may involve hearing their "problem" or "complaint" and helping them recognize that something different needs to be done to get a different result)
3. Look for strengths and abilities that can be used to make a desired change
4. Encourage application in problematic situation, and
5. Leave the door open for possible follow-up.

If therapist and client are open to the possibilities, a lot can get done in one session – whether the meeting occurs by-appointment or as a walk-in. Most likely to benefit and be satisfied with SST are those who want to solve a specific problem; those less likely to benefit or be satisfied are those who want a continuous long-term relationship for ongoing support and personal exploration.

Consistent with the mindset of single session thinking and practice, SST is not just a rushed or truncated version of a longer therapy – it is a planned and deliberate one-at-a-time (OAAT) psychotherapeutic approach to addressing a client's concerns. As Alistair Campbell (2012, p. 16) noted:

> SST is not a therapeutic model in itself, and [...] almost any therapeutic orientation could be adapted to working in a single-session way. The key aspect of the general frame is to ensure that the client walks away from a single session with a plan about how to solve their problems, the confidence that they have the skills and resources available, and the knowledge that they can come back at any time for further work.

Hoyt, Young, and Rycroft (2021, p. 4) identify four common themes that cut across and underlie single session thinking and practice, no matter the context:

1. *Attitude*: treating the session "as if" it might be the only one and hence making the most of every encounter
2. *Accessibility*: responding in a timely manner without any unnecessary barriers
3. *Acting Now*: accepting that the best opportunity to address change is NOW, and
4. *Alliance*: asking what clients want to achieve by the end of the session so that the therapist and client can work collaboratively, in the here and now, toward that goal.

Cannistrà and Piccirilli (2018/2021, p. 5) also remind us:

> SST is more than just a method for therapists to integrate into their own approach or practice. It is a way of considering and conducting therapy that has significant epistemological, practical, and organizational consequences. [...] It leads us to reflect on important issues such as the patient's role in the care process; the role of the therapist; decisive factors for change; the theoretical and technical choices a clinician makes which determine a therapy's success or failure; the whole way we conceive a therapeutic session, therapy, and the goals of helping relationships such as psychotherapy; how we organize healthcare; and more.

Common Errors in SST

In 1990 (p. xvi) Moshe Talmon wrote:

> *Single-Session Therapy* [...] is not about how to condense five or twenty sessions into one; rather, it shows how to make what is already there a useful and positive therapeutic experience. The single-session-therapy approach is offered to patients and therapists who are ready and motivated to take care of business *now*, and it leaves the door open to what has become known as intermittent therapy throughout the life cycle.

As Windy Dryden (2022, p. 125) notes, it is a mistake to attempt to cram the work of several sessions into one session and call it SST. Attempting to do too much can actually backfire: "Less could be more: more could be less" (Hoyt & Cannistrà, 2023b, p. 163). Dryden (2017, p. 15) explains:

> While time is at a premium in SST, the most effective single-session therapists seem to take their time and don't rush the process. It is much more important to work at the client's pace and to help the person to stay focused on their major issue and the related goal/solution. If you rush the process you will tend to be focused more on what you should cover than on helping the client where they are.

Jeff Young (2018/2021, p. 175) concurs:

> Remember it is impossible to fit more than one session into a session. Don't try to talk faster, don't try to cover everything, don't try to squeeze your usual 6 sessions into one session. Simply make time your friend, prioritize, and collaborate with your client on how best to make use of whatever time you have available.

As does Martin Söderquist (2023, p. 62):

> It is impossible to do everything in one session. OAAT requires focus and concentration from both parts [therapist and client] and what is important can't wait until next time because the OAAT session is the only one. Information overload needs to be put aside, all descriptions of clients' history and background aren't need (no need for an archeological dig) and the therapist[s] have to lead and follow to make the session effective by staying in the present.

Along similar lines, Karen Story (2018, p. 217) quotes an old English proverb:

> One thing at a time and that done well
> Is a very good rule as many can tell.

Hoyt and Cannistrà (2021/2023b, p. 159) tongue-in-cheek write "Sometimes clients succeed despite therapists' efforts – but someone with irony deficiency[1] who follows these sardonic strictures will be well on their way to avoiding

---

1   According to the *Encyclopedia Britannica* (retrieved September 24, 2021), "The term *irony* has its roots in the Greek comic character Eiron. [...] The Socratic irony of the Platonic dialogues derives from this comic origin." Aristotle also recommended language that was not obvious and that contained an antithesis that required investigation, "for then there is a learning process or something

successful single session (or other brief) therapy" and then provide a discussion of "Common Errors in Single Session Therapy":

1. Tell yourself that you MUST do a one-session SST – not that SST is a "one-at-a-time" (OAAT) mindset.
2. Insist on exclusively using your favorite model of therapy.
3. Inform the client that they will only get "one shot" and interpret any questioning as "resistance."
4. Let the client know that you don't expect success in one session – at least not for them and their problem(s). Curb enthusiasm.
5. Disregard reality – "It works *in practice* O.K., but does it work *in theory?*" (O'Hanlon & Wilk, 1987, p. ix).
6. Keep the session goal vague to avoid client feeling they have achieved their aim – "It's a long day on the course if you don't know where the hole is."
7. Don't ask the person what they think is a good way to address the problem – when Shakespeare wrote "Our remedies oft in ourselves do lie" (in *All's Well that Ends Well*, Act I, Scene 1, line 218) he clearly wasn't burdened with trying to build a caseload and make a comfortable living).[2]
8. Don't stop when you're ahead – start another topic without enough time.
9. Avoid small steps. Don't encourage the client to apply what has occurred before booking another session.
10. Avoid feedback that indicates client feels abandoned or needs more sessions.
11. Ignore context, language, meaning, history, beliefs, intentions, or motivation.
12. Rub the client's culture the wrong way.
13. Think that "to completely resolve a problem" is the only goal of SST. Call them a "dropout," a "quitter," "in denial," or a "borderline" if they want to stop before you do. What do they know – who's got the advanced degree and who's paying whom? As Dryden (2017, p. 2) has noted, a wry

---

very like it" (Grube, 1989, p. 89). *Irony deficiency* (*Urban Dictionary*, retrieved online 24 September 2021) is "A common deficiency in which the brain cannot process humor that contains irony."

2   Nor when he wrote in *Macbeth* (Act V, Scene 3, lines 40–47):

> *Macbeth:* Canst thou not minister to a mind diseased,
> Pluck from the memory a rooted sorrow,
> Raze out the written troubles of the brain,
> And with some sweet oblivious antidote
> Cleanse the stuffed bosom of that perilous stuff
> Which weighs upon the heart?
> *Doctor:* Therein the patient
> Must minister to himself.

definition could be: "A dropout from therapy is someone leaving therapy before their therapist believes they should."

14. Eschew implementation, supervision, ongoing training, and administrative support.

But What about the Money?

Shakespeare and his theater troupe did need to keep selling tickets and filling seats. So, what about the money? How is someone to make a living if they only see clients one time? They'll always be needing new customers, and it may be hard to keep their schedule full. Length of treatment is determined by some admixture of the therapist's theory and mindset; the client's problems, resources, and goals; and money – how much the therapist wants to be paid and how much the client can afford. In addition to Jay Haley (1990) saying that the most important decision in the history of therapy was to charge by the hour, I am also reminded of Ambrose Bierce's (1906/1957, p. 36) cynical definition in *The Devil's Dictionary*: "*Diagnosis* A physician's forecast of disease by the patient's pulse and purse."

In *The First Session in Brief Therapy* (Budman, Hoyt, & Friedman, 1992, pp. 77–78), Moshe Talmon was asked and answered:

QUESTION: How are we to make a living providing successful SST?

TALMON: When you recall that the majority of people with psychological problems never go to see a therapist, you may realize that there are many, many more people who can be helped by us. If being helped by a therapist is less expensive, more positive, and a safer experience than many of us were led to believe, then we are more likely to have our satisfied SST patients return for a checkup, another brief therapy, or even extended treatment sometime down the road – as well as referring many more patients to us.

SST (and other brief therapies) may be more popular in training programs and in clinics where staff are salaried than in the world of full-fee-for-service private practice, but this is changing. A recent feasibility study in Italy (Cannistrà et al., 2020) found very good acceptance for SST – even though the predominant view may still be toward long-term (psychoanalytic) treatment.[3] In 2018, an

---

3   The 4th International SST Symposium was held on November 10–12, 2023 in Rome (Cannistrà & Hoyt, in press; also see Cannistrà & Piccirilli, 2018/2021a). It's interesting to note that – in

article by Juno DeMelo in *O: The Oprah Magazine* (with a monthly circulation of 2.5 million) heralded SST. Dryden (2017) describes how, when a prospective client contacts him, he explains treatment options (SST, brief therapy, more extended therapy) and helps the client to make the appropriate choice for what the client needs. Talmon (in Hoyt, Rosenbaum, & Talmon, 1992, p. 78) also noted that if a patient comes to an HMO clinic seeking long-term, open-ended therapy, he often refers the patient to a highly reputable (and often expensive) fee-for-service practitioner, and "At times the patient returns with a better targeted and more realistic expectation. It is my observation that often all long-term therapy produces is simply more therapy."

One can have a mix of cases. Our primary ethical (including fiduciary) obligation is to serve the client's interest. I expect that if we provide informed options and let the client choose, therapists offering SST will have plenty of grateful customers.

Importance of Training, Implementation, and Supervision

Single session thinking and practice require both learning and application. *Training and supervision* involve teaching and learning. *Implementation* is the process that turns plans and learning into actions in order to accomplish strategic objectives and goals. If implementation is forgotten, "good ideas" may appear but they do not come to fruition (Hoyt, Young, & Rycroft, 2021, p. 339).

In *The First Session in Brief Therapy* (Budman et al., 1992, pp. 77–78), my SST co-originators and I had the following conversation:

QUESTION: It seems that doing SST would be an ideal model for training new clinicians. In other words, it is clearly confined to a particular time; it has a beginning, a middle, and an end; it requires the therapist to concentrate his or her thinking. Have you used it as a training model with new clinicians? How has this worked out?

HOYT: Training clinicians, whether beginners or experienced pros, to think about promoting change and empowering patients within a brief framework would be attractive, although

---

addition to SST – some of the most innovative developments in strategic and systemic brief therapy are from Italy, such as Giorgio Nardone's (e.g., Nardone & Watzlawick, 1990, 2005; Nardone & Salvini, 2018) work at Il Centro di Terapia Strategica d'Arezzo and the family therapy team of Mara Selvini Palazzoli and her colleagues in Milan (1978; Boscolo, Cecchi, Hoffman, & Penn, 1987; Boscolo & Bertrando, 1993; also see Loriedo & Vella, 1992; Hoyt, 2019b; Saladino, 2021).

SST can demand an eclectic innovativeness and flexibility that may require clinical experience and seasoning. [...] So far, the response has been enthusiastic and mostly positive, although some clinicians either find the SST approach too much of a stretch from their own theoretical predilections and/or mistakenly think we are claiming SST to be a panacea or cure-all or replacement for other forms of psychotherapy that may be required. We hope to teach clinicians ways of working efficiently and appropriately to help patients get unstuck, to make a shift or pivot. For most cases, the model of 'cure' is of dubious value and may interfere with the search for enhanced coping, new learnings, and growth. SST is not a 'cure.'

ROSENBAUM: Training clinicians in SST is more a question of inculcating a certain attitude than it is of passing on a set of techniques. This applies to both beginning and experienced clinicians. [...] Thus, we try to help clinicians approach each session with a certain openness to change in both themselves and the client, with curiosity and a willingness to let go and appreciate the experience that comes to them.

TALMON: New clinicians might be more open-minded and flexible and therefore require less 'unlearning' than we required ourselves as 'products' of many years of therapy for ourselves with deeply ingrained psychodynamic 'frames of mind.' On the other hand [...] new clinicians may be too anxious and too insecure in their knowledge to effectively and *selectively* employ SST.

Supervision involves one person (or more) looking over and instructing the work of another in order to help the latter improve his or her ability and performance. Several authors have discussed single-session supervision. Hoyt (1991/1995) notes parallel processes that may occur between therapist-client and supervisor-therapist; John Miller, Dai Xing, Hu Yaorui, and Xu Yilin (2021) describe teaching a seven-step protocol for Single Session Team Family Therapy; Joanna Bedggood (2018) enumerates various skills that prepare interns and new therapists for walk-in counseling; Luca Modenesi (in Torricelli, 2021, pp. 141–144) describes single-session clinical supervision in a trans-cultural setting; and Sandy Harper-Jaques (2018), based on her 10 years of experience, presents a "road map" for supervision of single-session walk-in therapists. Here are a couple of other reports:

- Hoyt and Robert Goulding (1989/1995) describe a two-part single session for the resolution of a transference-countertransference impasse using Gestalt/transactional analysis techniques in supervision. After a didactic (explanatory) portion, the supervisee said he still felt "stuck" and needed to "clarify" his position and so volunteered for an experiential process (1995, p. 246, emphasis in original).

Therapist (MFH):	I 'understand' it intellectually, drawing little circles and all that [alluding to T.A. models of Parent-Adult Child in transference-countertransference reactions], but somehow, I want to make it more *real*, reify it. [...] I feel like it's just happening, that I'm falling into it, even though I know I'm somehow activating it. I don't know what to do with this.
Supervisor (RLG):	Well, I do. Take your projection about your client and *be* it. [...] Just what you said about him, claim for yourself, because that's where you're stuck.

They then engaged in a 20-minute process (see original report for transcript and commentary) in which the supervisor directed a basic Gestalt exercise to own one's projections. At the conclusion, the therapist happily declared: "Yeah! That makes very real those circles!" In their closing discussion, the authors comment on the combined impact of both the didactic and experiential components to help the supervisee find the power within himself (and not primarily in a supervisor).

- Pam Rycroft (2018, in press) also describes parallels. She notes (2018, pp. 348–349) that, when "capturing moments" in supervision "There is also a musical analogy in the three-part sonata form."[4] [...] Using a *single session supervision* (SSS) case example, she illustrates that (2018, p. 364)

Just as SST considers each therapy session a whole therapy, SSS is a microcosm of supervision, with a beginning (Exposition) which includes a contracted agreement about what to focus on and how; a middle (Development) section, where the main theme is further developed,

---

4 For another example of a musical motif, see Rosenbaum and Bohart (2007). Also see Hoyt and Rosenbaum (2018) regarding use of a consolidating summary "coda" (akin to a musical ending) to provide a closing perspective in SST; and discussion in Chapter 4 (p. 112) regarding conceptualizing a traumatic memory as a prolonged fermata, a "long pause" (hyphen) rather than a "full stop" (period).

and new themes and variations explored; and the final (Recapitulation) section, with a return to the main theme, progress reviewed and further steps anticipated.

Implementation involves organizational and administrative arrangements, which may vary from place to place depending on intake systems, staffing, insurance, funding, community resources, etc. See discussions about the value of the walk-in SST/OAAT option in Chapter 3 and the importance of cross-cultural appropriateness for implementation in Chapter 5. Some valuable, overlapping general ideas for implementing SST are also available in the following:

- Young, Rycroft, and Weir (2014), based on their experience at The Bouverie Centre at La Trobe University in Melbourne, Australia, advise the following practical strategies for engaging practitioners, managers, CEOs, and funders:

  - Articulate a rationale for change. What's the problem and how can SST address this problem?
  - SST needs to fit with practitioner values and the philosophy of the host organization
  - Link SST to existing organizational processes, procedures, policy, and strategic directions
  - Get champions, managers, and leaders on side [aligned and working together]
  - Create an implementation team, an implementation process and plan
  - Provide good short-term training *and* long-term support
  - Provide resources to support implementation – time, technical support, processes
  - Use evaluation, numbers, and feedback systems
  - Plan for sustainability from the start.

They also offer and discuss these additional practical tips for implementing SST:

- Use agencies' existing client contact data
- Present the positives and negatives of introducing SST to everyone involved
- Use good timing – there may be competing projects, financial difficulties, etc. that can make it hard or impossible to introduce new practices.

- Suzanne Fuzzard (2021, in press; also see McDonald, Hickey, & Wyder, 2021; Renkin, Alexander, & Wyder, 2021) describes the experience of successfully embedding single session family consultation (SSFC – see Chapter 4, pp. 71–72) in a national youth mental health service in Australia. She notes and discusses (pp. 134–135) six reasons why she thought SSFC was so ideal:

  1. SSFC offered a framework in which clinicians could still use their trained models and skills when working with young people and families.
  2. It was not promoted as "family therapy" but rather as a meaningful consultative family meeting to provide timely focused assistance concerning the goals of the young person and family members.
  3. It is a framework that is do-able and very teachable to workers from a variety of professional backgrounds, and it could be modified for online delivery.
  4. Outcomes are measurable – client satisfaction being the overall aim.
  5. Since getting the whole family together can be logistically challenging, trying to have a *single* session seemed more achievable for many families and practitioners. Offering a *one-off* gave the opportunity to try it out without any further "strings attached."
  6. It enabled implementation sites to position themselves as services that worked meaningfully with families without identifying themselves as specialist family therapy services and risking clinicians worrying that they were working outside of their scope of practice.

- Alexandra Robinson, Grace Harvey, Molly McDonald, and Turi Honegger (2021) describe their experience introducing and implementing Single Session Therapy at a university counseling center in Santa Barbara, California. When they were first attempting to integrate SST with existing structures and organizational culture, even though they provided training on SST to the whole agency, they encountered significant clinician resistance that focused on worries that SST might not be culturally sensitive for traditionally underrepresented and underserved populations and

  the misconception that the model is an abbreviated substitute for regular therapy rather than a deliberate therapy intervention developed intentionally and based on worldwide data on the benefits of SST [...] Following suit from single session pioneers Hoyt and Talmon (2014, p. 4, italics added), the implementation team realized that the agency needed more information '*to view each encounter as a whole, complete in itself*' [p. 144].

They report that by continuing to engage with staff and leadership about existing research conducted in other agencies and by disseminating preliminary data about outcomes and case examples gathered at their clinic, SST gradually has been more embraced by the staff as evidenced by a growing SST team and a steady flow of referrals.

Robinson et al. note that to empower student-clients to be engaged in planning their treatment, a referring screener might say (p. 145):

A lot of people find that just one session is enough for them. You could choose to work on your concern with a Single Session appointment, which is a stand-alone meeting with a therapist focused solely on your goal, and it would be scheduled within a week. If you're interested in this option, I can tell you more.

For interested students, the screener will then further describe the format of the session and support them with identifying their goal for the session (p. 146):

The first 30 minutes of the session is the time when you and the therapist discuss what has been going on and what you are hoping to get help with. Then, there is a break in the session for 10–15 minutes during which time the therapist will consult with a team of therapist and brainstorm recommendations for you based on your goals. The remainder of the time is used to review the team's ideas with you and hopefully you will find some of the team's ideas helpful!

Likely Future Trends

These developments seem likely (Hoyt & Dryden, 2018; Dryden, 2021):

- More SSTs, by appointment and by walk-in
- More clinics offering SST
- More use of the Internet for providing single sessions – both for online ("telehealth") person-to-person SST and counseling and for the exciting low-intensity Single Session Interventions (SSIs) that Bennett, Myles-Hooton, Schleider, and Shafran (2022) and Schleider (2024) have been developing as part of "democratizing access to psychological therapies" (Singla, Schleider, & Patel, 2023)

- More publications, more conferences, and more trainings
- More research, including which groups and problems respond best to which approaches, and what actually happens – what are the "active ingredients" that make SST effective?
- More attention to cultural nuances, including greater appreciation of both Indigenous healing practices as well as those of nondominant ethnic-racial groups and other minorities (e.g., LGBTQ+) as part of much needed greater social justice
- More focus on approaches that emphasize client strengths and competencies, and how clients construe and construct – and revise – their personal psychological realities.

Alistair Campbell (2012, p. 24) writes:

> One of the major problems with most therapeutic process studies is the huge amount of data and the multiplicity of processes that have to be tracked. The circumscribed nature of the single session (lasting an hour or two) would radically reduce the complexity of any process study. It should be quite straightforward to explore a range of specific and nonspecific process factors that can be associated with positive outcomes over both short- and long-term timeframes. This seems to me a natural next step, rather than just repeating the same path to 'proving' that there is an effect. The really more interesting questions are: What is happening in a single session that is leading to change? Are these things happening in the first session of multisession therapies? If so, do they lead to change that is not being recognized or tapped? But also: Is the change that happens in a single-session modality specific? Does the therapeutic framework matter or does this just provide a structure for a focused change?[5]

SST is a common, effective, flexible, increasingly recognized and important component in the landscape of mental health service delivery. It is consistent with contemporary social and healthcare trends toward shorter waiting lists and lower costs, as well as the drive toward a more general do-it-yourself (DIY) attitude (Cannistrà & Cannistrà, 2021). It is not a panacea and not a replacement for other mental-health resources (which need additional

---

5   For some studies of SST processes, see Stiles et al. (2006), Ozaki (2017), Perdomo (2017), Matthews (2018), Fullen (2020), and Henneberry (2022). For more on harnessing the Single Session Intervention (SSI) approaches to promote scalable implementation of evidence-based practices in healthcare, see Schleider and Beidas (2022) and Bennett et al. (2022).

funding in a humane society) but will be a valuable and expanding part of the range of available therapy services.

Use of Single-Session/OAAT Thinking in Nonclinical Situations

Although the focus of this book is on single session therapy and the application of single session thinking and practice in clinical situations, single session thinking can also influence other endeavors. Chris Iveson, Evan George, and Harvey Ratner (2012), Ratner and Denise Yusuf (2015), and John Murphy (2023) give examples of one-session solution-focused coaching and school counseling. One might consult one time with a cooking instructor, a computer technologist, a vocational counselor, or a sports coach (see Pitt, Thomas, Lindsay, Hanton, & Bawden, 2015) – they would ascertain what skills you already have, what you're looking for, and try to assist you in getting there – without necessarily expecting another meeting. Visits to the plant nursery or home improvement center are usually one-at-a-time – they're complete unto themselves, until the next round. When we visit a restaurant, the meal has a beginning, middle, and end (appetizers, main dishes, dessert). Like with SST, it's a one-and-done and we might return sometime if we like what we got. Lots of meetings and presentations are also OAAT – there will be an agenda and perhaps action plans, but it's a one-time event. Indeed, one can teach an SST workshop (Hoyt, 2023) – or write a book! – using SST thinking. The medium mirrors the message – introduction and alliance, identification of goals and learning objectives, useful attitudes and mindset, consideration of existing skills and offering some new ones, encouragement of application, review, and planning next steps. Even in relationships that we hope or expect will be ongoing, single session thinking helps to focus on each encounter – what's today's topic/agenda, what needs to be done now whether we meet again or not? More generally, while long-range planning is useful and important, single session thinking and practice appreciates the meaning of the saying, "A journey of a thousand miles begins with a single step."

Take-Aways and Next Steps

The *APA Dictionary* (https://dictionary.apa.org/single-session-therapy; retrieved September 11, 2020) gives the following definition:

Single Session Therapy (SST): Therapy that ends after one session, usually by choice of the client but also as indicated by the type of treatment (e.g., Ericksonian psychotherapy, solution-focused brief therapy). Some clients claim enough success with one hour of therapy to stop treatment, although some therapists believe that this claim represents a flight into health or temporary relief from symptoms. Preparation for the session (e.g., by telephone) increases the likelihood of the single-session therapy being successful.

Various authors have suggested single session thinking and practice ideas to take with you when you see a client. Reviewing the following lists reveals single session mindsets, including Context of Competence attention to Alliance, Goals, and Resources. As you consider the different items, you may recognize aspects of the cases we have reviewed in the preceding chapters as well as have some ideas about how to adapt and apply the items to working with your own SST clients.

Bernard Bloom (1981, 1992, 2014), an early student of SST, offered 15 transtheoretical SST suggestions:

1. Identify a focal problem
2. Do not underestimate clients' strengths
3. Be prudently active
4. Explore, then present interpretations tentatively
5. Encourage expression of affect
6. Use the interview to start a problem-solving process
7. Keep track of time
8. Do not be overambitious
9. Keep factual questions to a minimum
10. Do not be overly concerned about the precipitating event
11. Avoid detours
12. Do not overestimate a client's self-awareness (i.e., don't ignore what may seem obvious)
13. Help mobilize social supports
14. Educate when clients appear to lack information
15. Build in a follow-up plan.

Arnie Slive and Monte Bobele (2011, in press b), champions of walk-in SSTs, delineate 11 principles:

1. The session is only one hour
2. Within that hour, we have a whole therapeutic session

3. Narrow the database to the immediate problem
4. Look for common factors
5. Be pragmatic
6. The session involves a consultation with other therapists
7. Focus on what the client wants from the session
8. Seek to understand the client's resources
9. Explore the client's previous attempts at a solution
10. Make use of the client's own motivations
11. Commend the client.

Windy Dryden (2017, 2019a, 2019b), working from an integrated single session/integrated cognitive-behavioral perspective, also articulates the main features of an SST/OAAT approach:

1. Celebrate the power of NOW and create a realistic expectation for the session
2. Ask the client how you may best help them
3. Develop an end-of-session goal
4. Agree on a focus for the session
5. Keep on track
6. Identify and utilize client strengths
7. Encourage the client to use environmental resources
8. Identify and utilize the client's previous attempts to deal with the problem
9. Negotiate a solution
10. Encourage the client to rehearse the solution
11. Encourage the client to reflect on the session, digest what they have learned, act on it, let time pass before seeking further help. As noted earlier, Dryden (2023 p. 14) has suggested the term *ONEplus Therapy* to emphasize that a client may come once "on the understanding that further help is available to the client on request."

Flavio Cannistrà (2018/2021, p. 93 and p. 112) outlines the phases of the Italian Center for Single Session Therapy method:

1. Pre-treatment: first impressions, questionnaire
2. Initial phase: establish the alliance, introduce single session, define problem in practical terms, clarify goal and identify priorities, ask for frequent feedback
3. Middle phase: investigate client's theory of change; identify resources and exceptions to the problem; explore dysfunctional behavior; give compliments, feedback, and suggestions; ask for feedback to make sure you are on track

4. Final phase: evaluate any relevant elements that may have been left out, prescribe homework, evaluate session, give instructions for "open door" return
5. Follow-up: request feedback sometime later and assess need for new appointment.

Pam Rycroft and Jeff Young, who have been conducting and researching SST at The Bouverie Centre in Melbourne since the early 1990s and have written extensively about it (e.g., Young & Rycroft, 1997; Rycroft & Young, 2014, 2021; Young, Rycroft, & Weir, 2014; Rycroft, 2018; Young, 2018), have taught thousands of clinicians and have developed an extensive online SST training program (see https://events.bouverie.org.au/sst). They offer a distillation of ten core elements for a single session:

1. Negotiate a client-led outcome
2. Establish the client's (or clients') priorities
3. Find a focus and talk about the most important things ("cut to the chase")
4. Check in with the client(s) at regular intervals
5. Interrupt respectfully when necessary (to help clients get what they want)
6. Make time your friend
7. Prepare to end well (reaching closure if not solution or resolution)
8. Share your thoughts openly with clients
9. Leave the door open (an "open door" policy)
10. Listen to client voices (follow up, seek feedback, and utilize it).

The Joy of SST

There is joy in helping someone quickly, and I hope that *Single Session Therapy: A Clinical Introduction to Principles and Practices* will help you and your clients to share that experience. As psychologists, therapists, and students of mental health, we have an urge toward helping, healing, and love – the sooner, the better.

A therapist who is also a visual artist, Roberta Guzzardi, kindly handed me this drawing in October 2017 after I had co-taught (with Drs. Flavio Cannistrà and Federico Piccirilli) a two-day SST workshop in Rome sponsored by the Italian Center for Single Session Therapy. The rainbow of figures happily floating between my hands represents some of the SST cases I had presented, in which clients in one session had overcome issues involving grief, nightmares, anxiety, depression, and relationship problems.

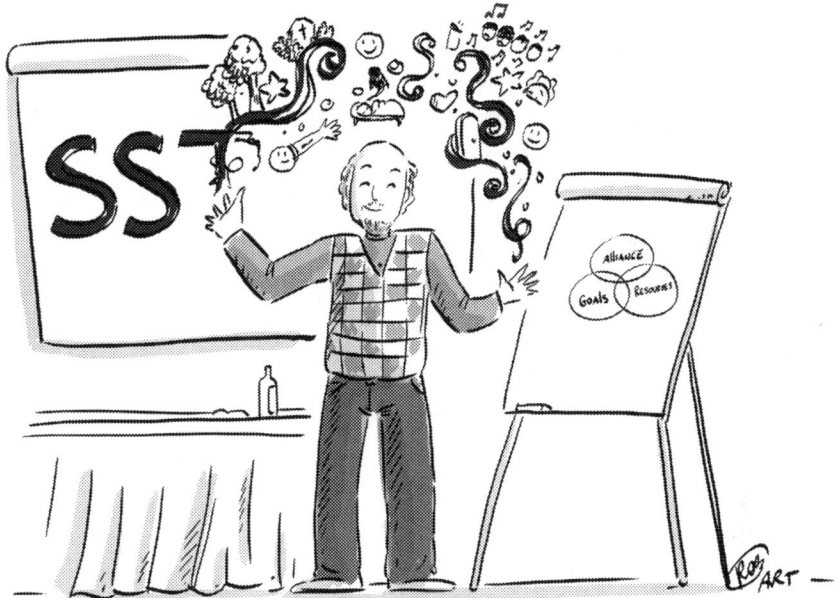

Figure 8.1 The Joy of SST

Source: by Roberta Guzzardi. ©2020. Used by permission.

What's Next?

Let's recall the learning objectives we started with (see Preface), and where in the preceding chapters information can especially be found:

1. List the basic features of brief therapy (see especially Chapter 1)
2. Describe the tasks and skills, including useful questions and specific techniques, associated with different phases of each session (pre-early, middle, late, follow-through) and with overall treatment (see especially Chapter 3)
3. Understand the Single Session Therapy/One-at-a-Time (SST/OAAT) mindset (see especially Chapter 2)
4. Analyze guidelines (indications, contraindications, steps) for SSTs (see especially Chapter 3)
5. Apply single-session intervention strategies to some of attendees' own clinical cases (see especially Chapters 4–7).

Long ago, Johann Wolfgang von Goethe (1749–1832) wrote: "All theory, dear friend, is gray, but the golden tree of life springs ever green" and (amplifying the call) "Knowing is not enough; we must apply. Willing is not enough; we must do." *So, how will you use single session thinking and practice?* We have considered various ideas, theories, strategies, methods, and presented a wide range of cases. Each person has their own experience base, skill set, and clinical context, so there is no one right answer – but what is your response, dear reader, to this question:

> *Suppose tonight, while you're sleeping, a miracle occurs – and when you wake up tomorrow you're an even more effective and efficient therapist than before – you're helping more clients in one session! How will you know? What will you be doing differently?*

Appendix A
Some SST Research Findings

A couple of years ago on a holiday card I wrote to an SST colleague:

'Twas the night before Christmas
And all through the Clinic
'SST? Let's see the data!'
Shouted the Cynic.
So the research team
Developed a scheme.
They surveyed and consulted
And got the best measures
And proved that SST
Can yield client-driven treasures.

Here is a sample of research studies demonstrating SST frequency and effectiveness. Additional citations can be found in Talmon (1990), Slive and Bobele (2011), Hoyt and Talmon (2014), Hoyt, Bobele, Slive, Young, and Talmon (2018b), Hoyt, Young and Rycroft (2021), Dryden (2017, 2019a, 2019b), Cannistrà and Pietrabissa (2021), Bennett, Myles-Hooton, Schleider and Shafran (2022), Kim, Ryu, and Chibanda (2023), Joseph (2023), and Pietrabissa (in press).

- Malan et al. (1968; also see Jacobson, 1968; Davanloo, 1978) at the Tavistock Clinic in London found that 51% of "untreated" neurotic patients who had only an intake interview showed less symptomatology; and Malan, Health, Bacal, and Balfour (1975), in a follow-up study, found that half of the 51% of "untreated" neurotic patients (25% of the total) also showed increased insight and personal responsibility and were found to have made important and enduring psychodynamic modifications. The "intake" had in effect been a one-session therapy.

- Mumford, Schlesinger, Glass, Patrick, and Cuerdon (1984), building on the work of Follette and Cummings (1967), Cummings and Follette (1976), and others, reviewed multiple replications of the finding of a significant reduction in medical utilization after a single session of psychotherapy. As Cummings and Follette (1976, p. 167) had written, "The finding that one session only, with no repeat psychological visits, could reduce medical utilization by 60 percent over the following five years, was surprising and totally unexpected." The "medical utilization offset phenomenon" is one of the ways mental healthcare can provide value to general medical services.[1]

- Silverman and Beech (1979) studied so-called "dropouts" at a community mental health center and concluded (p. 240) that "The notion that dropouts represent failure by the client or the intervention system is clearly untenable. Almost 80 percent of the clients interviewed reported that their problem(s) have been solved, 70 percent reported satisfaction with the services rendered, and the majority of client expectations of the center were met." Similar findings, that one-session "dropouts" actually had benefited and gotten what they wanted, are reviewed in Hoyt et al. (2018b, pp. 9–10). For example, Barrett, Chua, Crits-Christoph, Gibbons, and Thompson (2008) in a review that summarized the rate of stopping therapy after the first session as approximately 50%, appreciated that clients often achieve their goals in a relatively brief period of time, and although they framed much of their review in terms of "early withdrawal"

---

1   Many years later, Dr. Cummings (2013) was pleased to report that when Kaiser Permanente opened a new large medical center in Walnut Creek, California, the head of Kaiser said it was paid for by the savings in medical costs that resulted from their brief psychotherapy coverage. Nick also said that the head of Kaiser told Nick that they wanted to have a psychologist, not a medical doctor, be chief of mental health services, because otherwise the strong tendency would be to address emotional problems with medication rather than psychotherapy.

Another way that mental health services can make themselves an invaluable part of the overall medical enterprise is to help physicians and nurses manage those "difficult" patients who tend to wear out providers with demands that are ultimately at least partly psychological in nature (see Hoyt, 2008). Sometimes this can be accomplished in one session.

and "attrition," they recommended (p. 261) investigating "whether various types of clients benefit more or less from such [brief, ultra-brief, or single-session] treatments." Westmacott and Hunsley (2010) found that the most frequently reported reason for stopping therapy was feeling better. Swift and Greenberg (2012), in a meta-analysis of "premature discontinuation" in adult psychotherapy involving 669 studies and almost 84,000 clients, observed (p. 548) that "Therapist judgment has historically been considered the preferable classification [...] but this method depends on clinical judgment that can be biased and flawed." Similarly, a large-scale ($N = 8482$) multi-national World Health Organization survey reported 21.6% "dropping out" of mental-health treatment after the second visit and an overall 31.7% drop-out rate in which dropping-out was "defined as stopping treatment before the *provider* wanted" (Wells et al., 2013, p. 42, emphasis added). Unfortunately, they did not ask the *patients* why they had stopped treatment, and there was no mention of the possibility of successful single session (or other brief) therapy.

- Kellner, Neidhardt, Krakow, and Pathak (1992), at the University of New Mexico-Albuquerque, reported two single-session treatments (one involved exposure and relaxation training, the other involved authoring a new ending to the frightening scenario) that both significantly reduced recurring nightmares.

- Santor and Segal (2001) found that early positive psychotherapy responders were more likely to maintain gains. Gilboa-Schechtman and Shafar (2006) also found that early responders were more likely to maintain gains and hypothesized that findings of "the sooner, the better" were due to "remoralization" and a "successful integration of new cognitive, interpersonal, and behavioral habits into one's daily routine" (p. 380).

- Slive, MacLaurin, Oaklander, and Amundson (1995), Miller and Slive (2004), Miller (2008), Stewart et al. (2018), and McElheran (2021) reported high levels of client satisfaction for walk-in SSTs in several studies conducted at the Eastside Family Centre in Calgary, Canada. Similar results were reported by Josling and Cait (2018) and Lamsal, Stalker, Cait, Riemer, and Horton (2018) at KW Counselling Services in Kitchener, Canada. Additional affirmative proof-of-concept (feasibility) studies for walk-in family counseling in Australia have been reported by Hartley et al. (2023) and Moore et al. (in press).

- Hampson et al. (1999) at a child and adolescent mental health center in Canberra, Australia, found that 96% ($N = 70$) were satisfied with the scheduled SST and 88% reported the session helpful. Westwater,

Murphy, Handley, and McGregor (2020) reviewed subsequent research in child and adolescent mental and also conducted a mixed-methods (open questions and rating scales) investigation showing that over 50% of families find one SST encounter is enough with no need for further specialist input.

- McCambridge and Strang (2004), Daley and Zuckoff (1998), and Carroll, Libby, Sheehan, and Hyland (2001) found a single session of motivational interviewing to significantly reduce alcohol and drug abuse.

- Perkins (2006) reports the effectiveness of one session of therapy using an SST approach for children and adolescents with mental health problems at an Australian clinic; and Perkins and Scarlett (2008) document continuing benefits at 18-month follow-up assessment.

- Kutz, Resnick, and Dekel (2008) studied the effects of EMDR (Eye Movement Desensitization and Reprocessing) on acute distress syndrome following accidents and terrorist attacks in 86 patients and found 50% reported immediate fading of intrusive symptoms and general alleviation of distress after one session. Church (2014) reported several studies in which clinical EFT (Emotional Freedom Techniques, which involve tapping selected acupressure meridians) resulted in dramatic single-session improvements.

- Bhahot and Young (2009; reported in D'Alia, Giannetti, Bonadies, and Miele, 2021, p. 27; and Young, 2011a, 2011b) conducted a study of 409 clients seen at ROCK, a walk-in narrative therapy center for kids in Ontario, Canada. Parents and children completed a variety of questionnaires. Results indicated that clients felt significantly less worried, more competent as parents, more confident in their ability to solve or better manage the problem they had consulted about, and more aware of resources.

- In another study, Young and Bhanot-Malhotra (2014; see K. Young, 2018, pp. 66–68) evaluated the outcomes from a sample of single-session walk-in clinics across Ontario, Canada, that primarily use narrative therapy practices to serve children and youth. A total of 352 clients completed both pre-session and post-session measures, with 70 clients also completing three-month post-session measures. Results indicated that clients experienced a number of positive outcomes, including increased awareness about their own skills and ideas about how to solve the problem/issue that had brought them to therapy (with 80% having "aha moments" of discovery/realization), improvement in coping and perceptions of the problem as being less severe and/or frequent, and a high level of therapeutic alliance between clients and therapists.

- Kashdan, Adams, Read, and Hawk (2012) found in a randomized clinical trial that one session of exposure therapy yielded superior results. Similar one-session positive results were reported by Basoglu, Salcioglu, and Livanou (2007) for people experiencing PTSD after the 1999 Turkish earthquake. Nuthall and Townsend (2007) also reported a CBT-based early single-session intervention to be effective in preventing panic disorder.

- Walton and Cohen (2011) found improved long-term academic and health outcomes of African-American college students by having them in one session read and deliver a narrative that framed social adversity in school as shared and short-lived, promoting the stress-inoculation buffering belief that such difficulties were common and transient aspects of the college-adjustment process rather than an indication of some personal deficit or race-specific lack of social belonging. As the authors wrote (pp. 1450–1451): "Changing subjective construal is a fruitful avenue for intervention because many events are ambiguous and amenable to multiple interpretations. Moreover, a change in construal can become self-reinforcing. Students who feel confident in their belonging may experience the social world in a way that reinforces this feeling. They may initiate more relationships and thus obtain more opportunities for belonging and growth. Brief interventions that shore up belonging can thus promote performance and well-being even long after their delivery." In other words, a brief/single-session intervention can set off a salutary positive feedback loop, a virtuous (not vicious) cycle (Wender, 1968).

- Simon, Imel, Ludman, and Steinfield (2012; also see Scamardo, Bobele, & Biever, 2004) asked "Is dropout after a first psychotherapy visit always a bad thing"? and examined the survey responses at a group health plan of 2666 members, 906 (34%) of who did not return and found that (a) therapists and patients can form a good therapeutic alliance in one visit, and (b) those who did not return were more likely to report the most favorable and the least favorable outcomes. The authors conclude "Failure to return after an initial psychotherapy visit can represent successful and satisfying treatment. Systematic outreach and outcome assessment are necessary to identify the patients who drop out of therapy after unsuccessful and unsatisfying treatment."

- Hymmen, Stalker, and Cait (2013) reviewed seven studies of walk-in SST and found "that the SST has been sufficient from the clients' perspective approximately 60.9% of the time, which is remarkably similar to the 58.6% that Hoyt et al. (1992) reported 20 years ago." They noted (p. 1) that "The findings suggest that the majority of clients attending either previously scheduled or walk-in SST find it sufficient and helpful. The studies imply that this model of service delivery leads to perceived improvement in presenting problems in general, and on specific measures of variables such as depression, anxiety, distress level and confidence in parenting skills." Common themes of what walk-in SST clients considered most helpful include: receiving helpful advice about the problem, having the opportunity to talk about the problem and feel supported, being referred to other resources, and immediate accessibility of the walk-in service. The authors also note that "In fact, we have found no advocates of SST who claim this model is sufficient or even appropriate for all clients."

- Carey, Tai, and Stiles (2013) report data from Alice Springs, Australia, supporting the "effective and efficient" practice of allowing clients to call for appointments when wanted rather than having regularly scheduled visits. They also found that 25 of 92 studied patients chose to attend for a single session (even though more were available).

- Ollendick et al. (2009; also see Davis, Ollendick, & Ost, 2012) conducted a randomized clinical trial for 196 American and Swedish young people diagnosed with a spider phobia. Ollendick and Davis (2013) provide a brief historical overview and description of cognitive-behavioral one-session treatment (OST) for specific phobias in children and adolescents, and then systemically describe eight studies (conducted in Australia, Austria, the Netherlands, the US, and Sweden) that have examined its efficacy in youth aged between 7 and 17 years. They found considerable evidence that OST is generally effective across phobia subtypes and for both boys and girls and concluded that OST is a highly effective intervention for the treatment of specific phobias in children and adolescents.

- Harper-Jaques and Foucault (2014) assessed 98 clients who completed questionnaires one month after being seen at the walk-in service at the South Calgary (Canada) Health Centre and found high satisfaction, lower distress, and increased hope; moreover, 44% reported that SST was adequate.

- Schleider and Weisz (2017) assessed the effects of single session interventions (SSIs) for youth psychiatric problems, synthesizing findings from 50 randomized-controlled trials (10,508 youths were involved). Effect sizes (ES) varied by several moderators, including target problem: ESs were largest for anxiety (0.56) and conduct problems (0.54) and weakest for substance abuse. Findings support the promise of SSIs for certain youth psychiatric problems and the need to clarify how, to what degree, and for whom SSIs effect lasting change. For more on harnessing the single-session intervention approach to promote scalable implementation of evidence-based practices in healthcare, see Schleider and Beidas (2022), Bennett, Myles-Hooton, and Schleider (2022, 2024).

- Nardone and Salvini (2018) wrote: "From a strategic point of view [...] one can guide the patient to discover new perceptions that determine new reactions to the problem right from the first session. In so doing, we subtly introduce a chain reaction of changes: knowing through changing [pp. 23–24] [...] By leading the first session this way over the past four years, we found that 69–70% of patients had their symptoms reduced to zero between the first and the second session. These results are reflective of the majority of the psychopathologies treated with this model." [p. 27]

- Aafjes-van Doorn and Sweeney (2019) conducted a systematic literature search that resulted in 35 identified quantitative studies on the effect of initial therapy contacts. Although there was considerable variability in therapy format and various methodological limitations, qualitative synthesis of the effectiveness results suggested that a significant proportion of patients reported benefits, including symptom change. This positive effect was especially clear when compared to no-treatment controls and appeared to be maintained at follow-up.

- The annual report from the Center for Collegiate Mental Health (CCMH, 2019, p. 15) also reported that "The most common number of appointments per client/per year is one (1)."

- Kachor and Brothwell (2020) implemented and evaluated an SST pilot project in a youth community-based mental health and addiction clinic in Saskatchewan, Canada. Of the 179 youth/families that were reached for follow-up phone call (p. 52), "every client/family that was seen for SST reported that the single session had been helpful in some way. Comments reported ranged from the issue being completely resolved [37%], and there was no longer a need for services, to the session was helpful but further therapy was still requested [63%]." Significant clinical improvements in measures of anxiety, depression, and well-being were documented as well as reduced wait times.

- Cannistrà, Piccirilli, Pietrabissa, et al. (2020) examined the incidence and clients' experience of SST in Italy. In one study, they surveyed 476 traditional (not intentionally SST) clients and found that 26% elected to have a single session; in a second study, 85 consecutive patients who voluntarily asked for SST were assessed 1–3 weeks after consultation and 44 out of the 85 (52%) considered one session to be enough, as they felt better or much better and chose not to attend further sessions. Of the 41 clients who asked for a second session, 33 (80.5%) indicated that the first session was not enough and 8 (19.5%) wanted to address a new problem.

The authors concluded that these results converge with previous international studies and that they provide encouragement for the use of SST in both private and public psychological services to address the demand for timely mental health services in Italy. They also noted that further research is needed to support the efficacy of SST and to evaluate its cost-effectiveness.

- Bertuzzi et al. (2021) conducted a systematic review of the available evidence of the efficacy of SST on anxiety disorders in both youth and adults. They identified 18 reports based on rigorous inclusion criteria. SST was found superior to no treatment in reducing anxiety symptoms, and similar results were observed while comparing SST to multi-treatment sessions. The findings support the benefits of SST in enhancing cognitive, behavioral, and psychological outcomes in both youth and adults suffering from anxiety disorders across treatment conditions and approaches. The authors call for further research to quantify the cost-effectiveness of SST and to deepen knowledge of effective treatment ingredients.

- Robinson, Harvey, McDonald, and Honegger (2021) gathered data at the end of each SST ($n = 195$) at the University of California Santa Barbara Counseling and Psychological Services and found pre-session distress levels with a mean of 7.1 (on a 10-point scale) to be reduced post-session to a mean of 3.2.

- Darnall et al. (2021) found a single-session intervention of pain management skills to be superior to a rudimentary (control) single-session health education or to eight sessions of CBT for relief of anxiety and chronic lower back pain.

- Mulligan, Olivieri, Young, Lin, and Anthony (2022) used a convergent parallel mixed-methods design to assess the clinical effectiveness of SST for pediatric patients with neurological disorders and their families. The study comprised 135 participants, including patients, parents, and siblings across diverse neurological conditions. Scores of self-efficacy and anxiety in children, and distress and anxiety in adults, improved significantly after the SST. Notably, changes in anxiety in adults remained significant five to seven weeks after the SST. Seventeen participants participated in 12 semi-structured interviews. Participants described that SST (1) was a missing piece in ongoing clinical care, (2) illuminated existing strengths and resilience, and (3) effected a lasting impact beyond the single session.

- Söderquist (2023, pp. 128–133) reviewed research from various centers and also reported evidence from their Couple Counselling team in Malmö, Sweden, that indicates SST/OAAT to be helpful for reducing stress and increasing confidence in handling problems.

Appendix B

Single Session Therapy
Checklists/Exercises

The following three checklists can be used with the guideline questions presented in Chapter 3 to conduct training/practice exercises.

Checklist/Exercise 1: Pre-session Contact (Phone Call or Online)

Some questions to consider:

1. What's the problem? What is the situation now? (suicidal/homicidal/psychotic/medical)?
2. Who is the customer – who's most concerned?
3. What hidden agenda may there be? Other issues?
4. How and how soon does the client anticipate the problem will be solved?
5. How does client think therapy will be helpful in dealing with the problem?
6. What made client decide that now was the right time for therapy?
7. Do I need to consult with someone about this particular problem? Working with this ethnic group?
8. What assignment might be useful – to gather information, to recruit the patient's cooperation, to help shift their perspective? The Formula First

Session skeleton key question (de Shazer, 1985, 1988): "Between now and when we meet, I would like you to notice the things that happen to you that you would like to keep happening in the future. This will help me find out more about your goals and what you are up to." Another question: "Please give some thought to what you would like to accomplish in therapy, and how you will know if it's helping."

Checklist/Exercise 2: Beginning the Session (the Client Has Arrived)

Some tasks to accomplish:

1. Joining, connecting.
2. Orienting to purpose of meeting – help to solve a problem, help to determine the next steps you need to take, figure out what to do, identify how you can handle the situation, etc.
3. Mention availability of future sessions if needed and emphasize possibility of SST.
4. Recruit cooperation – work hard and figure out a solution; does that sound like something you want to do?
5. Assess current status – what has changed or been noticed since making appointment? Attempted solutions? How did that work?
6. Co-create achievable goals. General characteristics of well-formed goals (from de Shazer, 1991): (1) small rather than large; (2) salient to clients; (3) described in specific, concrete, behavioral terms; (4) achievable within the practical contexts of clients' lives; (5) perceived by clients as involving their hard work; (6) described as the "start of something" and not the "end of something"; and (7) treated as involving new behavior(s) rather than the absence or cessation of existing behavior(s).

Checklist/Exercise 3: Closing the Session (Finishing and Follow-Through)

Some items to address:

1. Giving feedback – emphasizing client's strengths and capacities.
2. Suggesting task or homework if indicated (have client design specifics)
3. Ask: How will you use this meeting? Next steps? Get specifics.
4. Leave door open. Invite follow-up, positive or negative.

References

Aafjes-van Doorn, K., & Sweeney, K. (2019). The effectiveness of initial therapy contact: A systematic review. *Clinical Psychology Review, 74*, 101786.

Adler, A. (1964). *The individual psychology of Alfred Adler.* Harper Perennial.

Ajmal, Y. (2001). Introducing solution-focused thinking. In Y. Ajmal & I. Rees (Eds.), *Solutions in schools* (pp. 10–29). BT Press.

Akerele, E., & Yuryev, A. (2017). Single session psychotherapy for humanitarian missions. *International Journal of Mental Health, 46*(2), 133–138.

Alexander, F., & French, T.M. (1946). *Psychoanalytic theory: Theory and applications.* Ronald Press.

American Psychological Association. (2017). *Multicultural guidelines: An ecological approach to context, identity, and intersectionality.* http://www.apa.org/about/policy/multiculturalguidelines.pdf.

Anderson, H. (1998). *Conversation, language and possibilities: A postmodern approach to therapy.* Basic Books.

Anderson, H., & Gehart, D. (Eds.). (2007). *Collaborative therapy: Relationships and conversations that make a difference.* Routledge.

Anderson, R.O. (1981). Shifting from external to internal provision of mental health services in a health maintenance organization. *Hospital and Community Psychiatry, 32*, 31.

Andreas, S. (2012a). Book review of D. Kahneman, *Thinking, fast and slow. The Milton H. Erickson Foundation Newsletter, 32*(3), 23.

Andreas, S. (2012b). *Transforming negative self-talk: Practical, effective exercises.* Norton.

Andreas, S. (2014). SST with NLP: Rapid transformations using content-free instructions. In M.F. Hoyt & M. Talmon (Eds.), *Capturing the moment: Single session therapy and walk-in services* (pp. 277–298). Crown House Publishing.

Armstrong, C. (2015). *The therapeutic "Aha!": 10 strategies for getting your clients unstuck.* Norton.

Appelbaum, S.A. (1975). Parkinson's Law in psychotherapy. *International Journal of Psychoanalytic Psychotherapy, 4*, 426–436.

Arnett, J.J. (2008). The neglected 95%: Why American psychology needs to become less American. *American Psychologist, 63*, 602–614.

Austad, C.S. (1996). *Is long-term psychotherapy unethical? Toward a social ethic in an era of managed care.* Jossey-Bass.

Baker, W. (1983). *Backward: An essay on Indians, time, and photography.* North Atlantic Press.

Bakewell, S. (2023). *Humanly possible: Seven hundred years of humanist freethinking, inquiry, and hope.* Penguin Press.

Balint, M. (1968). *The basic fault: Therapeutic aspects of regression.* Tavistock.

Bambling, M., King, R., Reid, W., & Wegner, K. (2008). Online counselling: The experience of counsellors providing synchronous single-session counselling to young people. *Counselling and Psychotherapy Research, 8*(2), 110–116.

Bandler, R., & Grinder, J. (1979). *Frogs into princes: Neuro linguistic programming* (S. Andreas, Ed.). Real People Press.

Bandler, R., & Grinder, J. (1982). *Reframing: Neuro-linguistic programming and the transformation of meaning* (S. Andreas & C. Andreas, Eds.). Real People Press.

Bandura, A. (1986). *Social foundations of thought and action: A social cognitive theory.* Prentice-Hall.

Bannink, F. (2011). *1001 solution-focused questions: Handbook for solution-focused interviewing* (2nd ed.). Norton.

Barbara-May, R. (2021). Collaborative first meetings with young people who have eating problems and their families. In M.F. Hoyt, J. Young, & P. Rycroft (Eds.), *Single session thinking and practice in global, cultural, and familial contexts: Expanding applications* (pp. 315–322). Routledge.

Barnes, M., Carruthers, P., & Gigovic, M. (2018). One...two...three ways to help you today: Therapeutic models in a single-session therapy program. In M.F. Hoyt et al. (Eds.), *Single-session therapy by walk-in or appointment* (pp. 175–185). Routledge.

Barrett, M.S., Chua, W.-J., Crits-Christoph, P., Gibbons, M.B., & Thompson, D. (2008). Early withdrawal from mental health treatment: Implications for psychological practice. *Psychotherapy: Theory, Research, Practice, Training, 45*(2), 247–267.

Barrett, R., Lapsley, H., & Agee, M. (2012). "But they only came once!" The single session in career counseling. *New Zealand Journal of Counseling, 32*(2), 71–82.

Barten, H.H. (1965). The 15-minute hour: A brief therapy in a military setting. *American Journal of Psychiatry, 122*, 565–567.

Basoglu, M., Salgioglu, E., & Livanou, M. (2007). A randomized controlled study of single-session behavioral treatment of earthquake-related post-traumatic stress disorder using an earthquake simulator. *Psychological Medicine, 37*(2), 203–213.

Bateson, G. (1979). *Mind and nature: A necessary unity.* Dutton.

Battino, R. (2000). *Guided imagery and other approaches to healing.* Crown House Publishing.

Battino, R. (2006). *Expectation: The very brief therapy book.* Crown House Publishing.

Battino, R. (2010). *Healing language: A guide for physicians, dentists, nurses, psychologists, social workers, and counselors.* Lulu.com.

Battino, R. (2014). Expectation: The essence of very brief therapy. In M.F. Hoyt & M. Talmon (Eds.), *Capturing the moment: Single session therapy and walk-in services* (pp. 393–406). Crown House Publishing.

Battino, R. (2020). *Using guided imagery and hypnosis in brief therapy and palliative care.* Routledge.

Battino, R. (2021, December). Guided Imagery Therapy (GIT) and Mirroring Hands Therapy (MHT): Brief, secret, and effective. *The Science of Psychotherapy*, 40–45.

Battino, R. (2022, November). Anabel: A case study. *The Science of Psychotherapy*, 48–53.

Battino, R. (2023). How to do Multiple Issue Psychotherapy (MIP). *The Science of Psychotherapy*, 11(6), 38–49.

Beaulieu, D. (2004). Lessons well learned: How to help your clients hold on to their gains. *Psychotherapy Networker*, 28(1), 27–28.

Bedggood, J. (2018). The first time: Teaching skills that prepare interns and new therapists for walk-in counseling. In M.F. Hoyt et al. (Eds.), *Single-session therapy by walk-in or appointment* (pp. 327–333). Routledge.

Bennett, S.D., Myles-Hooton, P., Schleider, J.L., & Shafran, R. (Eds.) (2022). *Oxford guide to brief and low intensity interventions for children and young people*. Oxford University Press.

Berenbaum, H. (1969). Massed time-limit psychotherapy. *Psychotherapy: Theory, Research and Practice*, 6, 54–56.

Berg, I.K. (1994). *Irreconcilable differences: A solution-focused approach to marital therapy*. Video. Norton.

Berg, I.K., & de Shazer, S. (1993). Making numbers talk: Language in therapy. In S. Friedman (Ed.), *The new language of change: Constructive collaboration in psychotherapy* (pp. 5–24). Guilford Press.

Berg, I.K., & Dolan, Y.D. (2001). *Tales of solution: A collection of hope-inspiring stories*. Norton.

Berg, I.K., & Miller, S.D. (1992). *Working with the problem drinker: A solution-focused approach*. Norton.

Bertuzzi, V., Fratini, G., Tarquinio, C., Cannistrà, F., Granese, V., Giusti, E. M., … & Pietrabissa, G. (2021). Single-session therapy by appointment for the treatment of anxiety disorders in youth and adults: A systematic review of the literature. *Frontiers in Psychology*, 12, article 721382. https://doi.org/10.3389/fpsyg.2021.721382.

Bierce, A. (1957). *The devil's dictionary*. Sagamore Press. (work originally published 1906)

Binfet, J.-T. (2017). The effects of group-administered canine therapy on university students' wellbeing: A randomized controlled trial. *Anthrozoös*, 30(3).

Biondo, N., & Gerber, N. (2020). Single-session dance/movement therapy for people with acute schizophrenia. *American Journal of Dance Therapy*, 42, 277–295.

Birkin, R. (2021). Single session approaches with infants: A collaborative single session model. In M.F. Hoyt, J. Young, & P. Rycroft (Eds.), *Single session thinking and practice in global, cultural, and familial contexts: Expanding applications* (pp. 192–201.). Routledge.

Bisson, J.I. (2003). Single-session early psychological interventions following traumatic events. *Clinical Psychology Review*, 23(3), 481–499.

Blake, W. (1966). *Augeries of innocence*. In G. Keynes (Ed.), *Blake: Complete writing with variant readings*. Oxford University Press. (Work originally published 1806.)

Bloom, B.L. (1981). Focused single-session therapy: Initial development and evaluation. In S.H. Budman (Ed.), *Forms of brief therapy* (pp. 167–216). Guilford Press.

Bloom, B.L. (ed.) (1992). Bloom's focused single-session therapy. In *Planned short-term psychotherapy: A clinical handbook* (2nd ed., pp. 97–121). Allyn & Bacon.

Bloom, B.L. (2001). Focused single session psychotherapy: A review of the clinical and research literature. *Brief Treatment and Crisis Intervention*, 1(1), 75–86.

Bloom, B.L. (2014). Foreword. In M.F. Hoyt & M. Talmon (Eds.), *Capturing the moment: Single session therapy and walk-in services* (pp. xv–xvi). Crown House Publishing.

Blymyer, D. (1991). The rapid resolution of auditory hallucinations. *Journal of Systemic Therapies*, 10(2), 1–5.

Bobele, M. (1987). Therapeutic interventions in life-threatening situations. *Journal of Marital and Family Therapy, 13*(3), 225–239.

Bobele, M. (1988). "Public policy in life-threatening situations": A reply. *Journal of Marital and Family Therapy, 14*(2), 139–141.

Bobele, M. (2019). On a small island off the coast of Texas. In M.F. Hoyt & M. Bobele (Eds.), *Creative therapy in challenging situations: Unusual interventions to help clients* (pp. 30–46). Routledge.

Bobele, M., Fullen, C., Houston, B., Martinez, A.M., Moffat, L., & Santos, J. (2018). Westside stories: Walk-in and single-session therapy in San Antonio. In M.F. Hoyt et al., *Single-session therapy by walk-in or appointment* (pp. 221–250). Routledge.

Bobele, M., López, S. S.-G., Scamardo, M., & Solórzano, B. (2008). Single-session/walk-in therapy with Mexican-American clients. *Journal of Systemic Therapies, 27*(4), 75–89.

Bobele, M., & Slive, A. (2014). One session at a time: When you have a whole hour. In M.F. Hoyt & M. Talmon (Eds.), *Capturing the moment: Single session therapy and walk-in services* (pp. 95–119). Crown House Publishing.

Bobele, M., & Slive, A. (2015). Walk-in psychotherapy: A new paradigm. *The Milton H. Erickson Foundation Newsletter, 35*(2), 9.

Bobele, M., & Slive, A. (2021). An open invitation to walk-in therapy: Opening access to mental health care. In M.F. Hoyt et al. (Eds.), *Single session thinking and practice in global, cultural, and familial contexts: Expanding applications* (pp. 54–65). Routledge.

Bonanno, G.A. (2021). *The end of trauma: How the new science of resilience is changing how we think about PTSD.* Basic Books.

Bond, F.W., & Dryden, W. (2002). *Handbook of brief cognitive behavior therapy.* Wiley.

Bordin, E.S. (1979). The generalizability of the psychoanalytic concept of the working alliance. *Psychotherapy: Theory, Research & Practice, 16*(3), 252–260.

Borges, J.L. (1964). A new refutation of time. In *Labyrinths: Selected stories & other writing* (pp. 217–234). New Directions. (Work originally published in Spanish in 1947.)

Boscolo, L., & Bertrando, P. (1993). *The times of time: A new perspective in systemic therapy and consultation.* Norton.

Boscolo, L., Cecchi, G., Hoffman, L., & Penn, P. (1987). *Milan systemic family therapy: Conversations in theory and practice.* Basic Books.

Bourdain, A. (2007). *Kitchen confidential: Adventures in the culinary underbelly* (rev. ed.). HarperCollins.

Boyd-Franklin, N. (2003). *Black families in therapy: A multisystems approach* (2nd ed.). Guilford Press.

Boyhan, P.A. (1996). Clients' perceptions of single session therapy consultations as an option to waiting for family therapy. *Australian and New Zealand Journal of Family Therapy, 17*(2), 85–96.

Boyhan, P.A. (2014). Innovative uses for single session therapy: Two case studies. In M.F. Hoyt & M. Talmon (Eds.), *Capturing the moment: Single session therapy and walk-in services* (pp. 157–175). Crown House Publishing.

Boyhan, P.A. (2021). Complex and challenging issues in SST: Reflections on the past and learnings for the future. In M.F. Hoyt, J. Young, & P. Rycroft (Eds.), *Single session thinking and practice in global, cultural, and familial contexts: Expanding applications* (pp. 173–181). Routledge.

Brehm, J. W. (1966). *A theory of psychological reactance.* Academic Press.

Breuer, J., & Freud, S. (1893–95). Studies in hysteria. In *Standard edition of the complete psychological works of Sigmund Freud* (vol. 2, pp. 1–319). Hogarth Press, 1955.

Budman, S.H. (1990). The myth of termination in brief therapy: Or, it ain't over until it's over. In J.K. Zeig & S.G. Gilligan (Eds.), *Brief therapy: Myths, methods, and metaphors* (pp. 206–218). Brunner/Mazel.

Budman, S.H., & Gurman, A.S. (1988). *Theory and practice of brief therapy*. Guilford Press.

Budman, S.H., & Hoyt, M.F. (1993). Active intervention in brief therapy and control-mastery theory: A case study. In R.A. Wells & V.J. Giannetti (Eds.), *Casebook of the brief psychotherapies* (pp. 21–26). Plenum.

Budman, S.H., Hoyt, M.F., & Friedman, S. (Eds.) (1992). *The first session in brief therapy*. Guilford Press.

Bundy, N. (2022). Time, complexity, and the meaning of help: A systematic review of people's experience of single-session therapy. *Journal of Systemic Therapies, 41*(2), 68–87.

Burns, D.D. (1980). *Feeling good: The new mood therapy*. William Morrow.

Burns, D.D. (2020). *Feeling great: The revolutionary new treatment for depression and anxiety*. PESI Publishing & Media.

Bundy, N. (2022). Time, complexity, and the meaning of help: A systematic review of people's experience of single-session therapy. *Journal of Systemic Therapies, 41*(2), 68–87.

Calvin, W.H. (1986). *The river that flows uphill: A journal from the Big Bend to the big brain*. Sierra Club Books.

Cameron, C. (2007). Single session and walk-in psychotherapy: A descriptive account of the literature. *Counselling and Psychotherapy Research, 7*(4), 245–249.

Campbell, A. (1999). Single session interventions: An example of clinical research in practice. *Australian and New Zealand Journal of Family Therapy, 20*(4), 183–194.

Campbell, A. (2012). Single-session approaches to therapy: Time to review. *Australian and New Zealand Journal of Family Therapy, 33*(1), 15–26.

Campbell, J. (1949). *The hero with a thousand faces*. Bollingen Foundation Press.

Cannistrà, F. (2019). A violent life: Using brief therapy "logics" to facilitate change. In M.F. Hoyt & M. Bobele (Eds.), *Creative therapy in challenging situations: Unusual interventions to help clients* (pp. 47–57). Routledge.

Cannistrà, F. (2021a). The Italian center for single session therapy method. In F. Cannistrà & F. Piccirilli (Eds.), *Single-session therapy: Principles and practice* (pp. 89–119). Giunti. (Published in Italian in 2018.)

Cannistrà, F. (2021b). The vital role of the therapist's mindset. In M.F. Hoyt, J. Young, & P. Rycroft (Eds.), *Single session thinking and practice in global, cultural, and familial contexts* (pp. 77–88). Routledge.

Cannistrà, F. (2022). The single session therapy mindset: Fourteen principles gained through an analysis of the literature. *International Journal of Brief Therapy and Family Science, 12*(1), 1–26.

Cannistrà, F., & Cannistrà, A. (2021). Single-session therapy: Reflections and perspectives on contemporary social and healthcare systems. In F. Cannistrà & F. Piccirilli (Eds.), *Single-session therapy: Principles and practice* (pp. 185–200). Giunti. (Published 2018 in Italian.)

Cannistrà, F., & Hoyt, M.F. (2020). The 9 logics beneath brief therapy interventions: A framework to help therapists achieve their purpose. *Journal of Systemic Therapies, 39*(1), 19–34.) An extended version appears in M.F. Hoyt & F. Cannistrà, *Brief therapy conversations: Exploring efficient intervention in psychotherapy* (pp. 135–156). Routledge, 2023.

Cannistrà, F., & Hoyt, M.F. (Eds.) (in press). *Single session therapies: Why and how one-at-a-time mindsets are effective.* Routledge.

Cannistrà, F., & Piccirilli, F. (2021a). *Single-session therapy: Principles and practices.* Giunti. (Published in Italian in 2018.)

Cannistrà, F., & Piccirilli, F. (2021b). *Terapia breve centrata sulla soluzione: Principi e pratiche* [*Solution-focused brief therapy: Principles and practices*]. Giunti. (Published in Italian.)

Cannistrà, F., & Piccirilli, F. (2021c). SST pre-treatment questionnaire. In *Single-session therapy: Principles and practice* (p. 201). Giunti. (Published in Italian in 2018.)

Cannistrà, F., Piccirilli, F., Pietrabissa, G., D'Alia, P.P., Giannetti, A., Piva, L., … Ghisoni, A. (2020). Examining the clinical efficacy and clients' experiences of single session therapy in Italy: A feasibility study. *Australian and New Zealand Journal of Family Therapy, 41*(3), 271–282.

Cannistrà, F., & Pietrabissa, G. (2021). Single-session therapy: Data and effectiveness. In F. Cannistrà & F. Piccirilli (Eds.), *Single-session therapy: Principles and practice* (pp. 33–48). Giunti.

Carey, T.A., Tai, S.J., & Stiles, W.B. (2013). Effective and efficient: Using patient-led appointment scheduling in routine mental health practice in remote Australia. *Professional Psychology: Research and Practice, 44*(6), 405–414.

Carlson, J. (2000). How to prevent relapse: Treatment strategies for long-term change. *Family Therapy Networker, 24,* 23 and 84.

Carroll, K.M., Libby, B., Sheehan, J., & Hyland, N. (2001). Motivational interviewing to enhance treatment initiation in substance abusers: An effectiveness study. *American Journal on Addictions, 10,* 335–339.

Castelnuovo-Tedesco, P. (1986). *The twenty-minute hour: A guide to brief psychotherapy.* American Psychiatric Press.

Castenada, C. (1968). *The teachings of Don Juan: A Yaqui way of knowledge.* Washington Square Press.

Center for Collegiate Mental Health. (2020, January). *2019 Annual Report* (Publication No. STA 20–244). Penn State University.

Chang, J., & Phillips, M. (1993). Michael White and Steve de Shazer: New directions in family therapy. In S.G. Gilligan & R. Price (Eds.), *Therapeutic conversations* (pp. 95–111). Norton.

Chow, D. (2018). *The first kiss: Undoing the intake model and igniting the first sessions in psychotherapy.* Correlate Press.

Chubb, H., & Evans, E. (1985). "Therapy is not going to help": Brief family treatment of a character disorder. *Journal of Strategic and Systemic Therapies, 4,* 37–44.

Church, D. (2014). Clinical EFT (Emotional Freedom Techniques) as single session therapy: Cases, research, indications, and cautions. In M.F. Hoyt & M. Talmon (Eds.), *Capturing the moment: Single session therapy and walk-in services* (pp. 299–324). Crown House Publishing.

Clements, R., McElheran, N., Hackney, L., & Park, H. (2011). The Eastside Family Centre: 20 years of single-session walk-in therapy – where we have been and where we are going. In A. Slive & M. Bobele (Eds.), *When one hour is all you have: Effective therapy for walk-in clients* (pp. 109–127). Zeig, Tucker, & Theisen.

Cohen, B., Daley, G., & Northe, V. (2021). Single session therapy for those affected by gambling: Listening to clients and their therapeutic counselors. In M.F. Hoyt, J. Young, & P. Rycroft (Eds.), *Single session thinking and practice in global, cultural, and familial contexts: Expanding applications* (pp. 296–304). Routledge.

Collins, B.E., & Hoyt, M.F. (1972) Magnitude of inducement, consequences, and responsibility choice: An integration and extension of the "forced compliance" literature. *Journal of Experimental Social Psychology,* 1972, 8, 558–593. Reprinted as *Warner Publication Module,* No. 243, 1973. Reprinted (in German) in *Sozialpsychologie I,* 1979, Wissenschaftliche Buchgesellschaft, Darmstadt. Reprinted (in Japanese) in *Handbook of Experimental Social Psychology 5,* 1988, Seishin Shobo, Tokyo.

Connie, E.E. (2012). *Solution building in couples therapy.* Springer.

Connie, E.E., & Froerer, A.S. (2023). *The solution focused brief therapy diamond: A new approach to SFBT that will empower both practitioner and client to achieve the best outcomes.* Hay House.

Constantine, L.L. (1978). Family sculpture and relationship mapping techniques. *Journal of Marital and Family Therapy,* 4(2), 13–23.

Cooley, C. H. (1902). *Human nature and social order.* C. Scribner's Son.

Cooper, L.F., & Erickson, M.H. (1959). *Time distortion in hypnosis: An experimental and clinical investigation.* Williams & Watkins. (Reissued 2002 by Crown House Publishing.)

Cooper, M., & McLeod, J. (2007). A pluralistic framework for counselling and psychotherapy: Implications for research. *Counselling and Psychotherapy Research* 7(3), 135–143.

Cooper, S.J. (2024). *Brief narrative practice in single-session therapy.* Routledge.

Cooper, S.J. (in press). Brief narrative practices in single-session therapy. In F. Cannistrà & M.F. Hoyt (Eds.), *Single session therapies: Why and how one-at-a-time mindsets are effective.* Routledge, forthcoming.

Cooper, S., & "Ariane." (2018). Co-crafting take-home documents at the walk-in. In M.F. Hoyt et al. (Eds.), *Single-session therapy by walk-in or appointment* (pp. 260–269). Routledge.

Corey, G. (2017). *Theory and practice of counseling and psychotherapy* (10th ed.). Cengage Learning.

Cornish, P.M. (2020). *Stepped care 2.0: A paradigm shift in mental health.* Springer.

Costa, C.D.N. (Ed.) (2005). *On the shortness of life: Life is long if you know how to use it.* Penguin.

Courtnage, A. (2020). Hoping for change: The role of hope in single-session therapy. *Journal of Systemic Therapies,* 39(1), 49–63.

Cowmeadow, P. (1995). Very brief psychotherapeutic interventions with deliberate self-harmers. In A. Ryle (Ed.), *Cognitive analytic therapy: Developments in theory and practice* (pp. 55–66). Wiley.

Coyne, J.C. (1985). Toward a theory of frames and reframing. *Journal of Marital and Family Therapy,* 11, 337–344.

Coyne, J. C. (1987). The concept of empowerment in strategic therapy. *Psychotherapy: Theory, Research, Practice, Training,* 24(3), 539–545.

Crenshaw, W. (2004). *Treating families and children in the child protective system.* Brunner-Routledge.

Cummings, N.A. (2000). The single session misunderstanding. In *The collected papers of Nicholas A. Cummings. Vol. 1: The value of psychological treatment* (p. 77; J.L. Thomas & J.L. Cummings, Eds.). Zeig, Tucker, & Theisen.

Cummings, N.A. (2013). Psychotherapy's soothsayer. In M.F. Hoyt (Ed.), *Therapist stories of inspiration, passion, and renewal: What's love got to do with it?* (pp. 58–66). Routledge.

Cummings, N.A., & Follette, W.T. (1976). Brief therapy and medical utilization. In H. Dorken et al. (Eds.), *The professional psychologist today.* Jossey-Bass.

Cummings, N.A., & Sayama, M. (1995) *Focused psychotherapy: A casebook of brief, intermittent psychotherapy through the life cycle.* Brunner/Mazel.

D'Alia, P.P., Giannetti, A., Bonadies, S., & Miele, R. (2021). Single session therapy: Past and present. In F. Cannistrà & F. Piccirilli (Eds.), *Single-session therapy: Principles and practice* (pp. 13–31). Giunti.

Daley, D.C., & Zuckoff, A. (1998). Improving compliance with the initial outpatient session among discharged inpatient dual diagnosis clients. *Social Work, 43,* 470–473.

Darnall, B. D., Roy, A., Chen, A. L., Ziadni, M. S., Keane, R. T., You, D. S., ... & Mackey, S. C. (2021). Comparison of a single-session pain management skills intervention with a single-session health education intervention and 8 sessions of cognitive behavioral therapy in adults with chronic low back pain: A randomized clinical trial. *JAMA Network Open, 4*(8), e2113401. https://doi.org/10.1001/jamanetworkopen.2021.13401

Dattilio, F.M. (Ed.) (1998). *Case studies in couple and family therapy: Systemic and cognitive perspectives.* Guilford Press.

Davanloo, H. (1978). Short-term dynamic psychotherapy of one or two sessions duration. In H. Davanloo (Ed.), *Basic principles and techniques in short-term dynamic psychotherapy* (pp. 307–326). Spectrum Publications.

Davis, T.E. III, Ollendick, T.H., & Öst, L.-G. (Eds.) (2012). *Intensive one-session treatment of specific phobias.* Springer Science + Business Media.

DeJong, P, & Berg, I.K. (1997). *Interviewing for solutions.* Brook/Cole.

Del Grande, C. (2023, November 10). *Setting the mindset of Single Session Therapy using a pre-session questionnaire: An experimental study.* Paper presented at 4th International Single Session Therapy Symposium, Rome.

DeMelo (2018, July). Bull's eye! One-and-done sessions give new meaning to the phrase targeted therapy. *O: The Oprah Magazine, 19,* 63–64 and 67.

Denborough, D. (2014). *Retelling the stories of our lives: Everyday narrative therapy to draw inspiration and transform experience.* Norton.

Denner, S., & Reeves, S. (1997). Single session assessment and therapy for new referrals to CMHTS. *Journal of Mental Health, 6*(3), 275–280.

de Shazer, S. (1985). *Keys to solution in brief therapy.* Norton.

de Shazer, S. (1988) *Clues: Investigating solutions in brief therapy.* Norton.

de Shazer, S. (1991a). Foreword. In Y.M. Dolan (Ed.), *Resolving sexual abuse: Solution-focused therapy and Ericksonian hypnosis for adult survivors* (pp. ix–x). Norton.

de Shazer, S. (1991b). *Putting difference to work.* Norton.

de Shazer, S. (1993). Creative misunderstanding: There is no escape from language. In S. G. Gilligan & R. Price (Eds.), *Therapeutic conversations* (pp. 81–90). Norton.

de Shazer, S., Dolan, Y., Korman, H., Trepper, T., McCollum, E., & Berg, I.K. (2007). *More than miracles: The state of the art of solution-focused brief therapy.* Routledge.

Dilley, J.W., Woods, W.J., Loeb, L., Nelson, K., Sheon, N., Mullan, J., et al. (2007). Results from a randomized controlled trial using paraprofessional counselors. *Journal of Acquired Immune Deficiency Syndromes, 44*(5), 569–577.

Dilley, J.W., Woods, W.J., Sabatino, L., Lihatsh, T., Adler, B., Casey, S., et al. (2002). Changing sexual behavior among gay male repeat testers for HIV: A randomized, controlled trial of a single-session intervention. *Journal of Acquired Immune Deficiency Syndromes, 30*(2), 177–186.

Doran, G. T. (1981). There's a S.M.A.R.T. way to write management's goals and objectives. *Management Review, 70*(11), 35–36.

Dreiblatt, I.S., & Weatherly, D. (1965). An evaluation of the efficacy of brief contact therapy with hospitalized psychiatric patients. *Journal of Consulting Psychology, 29*, 513–519.

Dryden, W. (2011). *Counselling in a nutshell* (2nd ed). Sage.

Dryden, W. (2016). *When time is at a premium: Cognitive behavioral approaches to single- session therapy and very brief couching*. Rationality Publications.

Dryden, W. (2017). *Single-session integrated CBT (SSI-CBT)*. Routledge.

Dryden, W. (2018). *Very brief therapeutic conversations*. Routledge.

Dryden, W. (2019a). *Single-session 'one-at-a-time' therapy: A rational-emotive behaviour therapy approach*. Routledge.

Dryden, W. (2019b). *Single-session therapy: 100 key points and techniques*. New York: Routledge.

Dryden, W. (2020). Single-session one-at-a-time therapy: A personal approach. *Australian and New Zealand Journal of Family Therapy, 41*(3), 283–301.

Dryden, W. (2021a) *Single-session therapy and its future: What SST leaders think*. Routledge.

Dryden, W. (2021b). Sign up, meet up, speak out: Single sessions in the context of meet-up groups. In M.F. Hoyt, J. Young, & P. Rycroft (Eds.), *Single session thinking and practice in global, cultural, and familial contexts: Expanding applications* (pp. 153–162). Routledge.

Dryden, W. (2021c). *Help yourself with single-session therapy*. Routledge.

Dryden, W. (2022). *Single-session therapy: Responses to frequently asked questions*. Routledge.

Dryden, W. (2023, Summer). What's in a name? What to call therapy where a client may come once. *InsideOut, 100*, 12–14.

Dryden, W. (in press). Bringing a single-session mindset to counseling in an online health service. In F. Cannistrà & M.F. Hoyt (Eds.), *Single session therapies: Why and how one-at-a- time mindsets are effective*. Routledge. forthcoming.

Duncan, B.L., Miller, S.D., Wampold, B., & Hubble, M. (2009). *The heart and soul of change: Delivering what works in therapy* (2nd ed.). APA Books.

Dunnachie, B., Isherwood, K., & Porter, S. (2021). Single session family consultation in Aotearoa New Zealand: Cultural considerations. In M.F. Hoyt, J. Young, & P. Rycroft (Eds.), *Single session thinking and practice in global cultural, and familial contexts* (pp. 234–244). Routledge.

Duvall, J., & Beres, L. (2011). *Innovations in narrative therapy: Connecting practice, training, and research*. Norton.

Duvall, J., Young, K., & Kayes-Burden, A. (2012). *No more, no less: Brief mental health services for children and youth*. www.windzcentre.com

Dylan, B. (1975). If you see her, say hello. Song on *Blood on the tracks* record album. Columbia Records.

Dylan, B. (2022). *The philosophy of modern song*. Simon & Schuster.

Eco, U. (1983). *The name of the rose*. Harcourt. (Work originally published in Italian as *Il nome della rosa* in 1980.)

Eisenthal, S., & Lazare, A. (1976a). Specificity of patients' requests in the initial interview. *Psychological Reports, 38*, 739–748.

Eisenthal, S., & Lazare, A. (1976b). Evaluation of the initial interview in a walk-in clinic: The patient's perspective on a "customer approach." *Journal of Nervous and Mental Disease, 162*, 169–176.

Elliott, A., Dokona, J., & von Doussa, H. (2021). Following the river's flow: A conversation about single session approaches with Aboriginal families. In M.F. Hoyt, J. Young, & P. Rycroft (Eds.), *Single session thinking and practice in global, cultural, and familial contexts* (pp. 213–222). Routledge.

Ellis, A. (1998). How rational emotive behavior therapy belongs in the constructivist camp. In M.F. Hoyt (Ed.), *The handbook of constructive therapies* (pp. 83–99). Jossey-Bass.

Ellis, A., & Dryden, W. (1987). *The practice of rational-emotive therapy*. Springer.

Ellis, A., & Joffe, D. (2002). A study of volunteer clients who experienced live sessions of rational emotive behavior therapy in front of a public audience. *Journal of Rational-Emotive and Cognitive-Behavior Therapy, 20,* 151–158.

Englar-Carlson, M. (2024). Series preface. In J.J. Murphy (Ed.), *Solution-focused therapy* (pp. ix–xiii). APA Books.

Epston, D. (1993). Internalized other questioning with couples: The New Zealand version. In S.G. Gilligan & R. Price (Eds.), *Therapeutic conversations* (pp. 183–189). Norton.

Erickson, M.H. (1954a). Pseudo-orientation in time as hypnotic procedure. *Journal of Clinical and Experimental Hypnosis, 2,* 261–283.

Erickson, M.H. (1954b). Special techniques in brief hypnotherapy. *Journal of Clinical and Experimental Hypnosis, 2,* 109–129.

Erickson, M.H. (1980). *Collected papers* (E.L. Rossi, Ed.). Irvington.

Erickson, M.H., & Rossi, E.L. (1979). *Hypnotherapy: An exploratory casebook*. Irvington.

Erickson, M.H., Rossi, E.L., & Rossi, S.I. (1976). *Hypnotic realities: The induction of clinical hypnosis and forms of indirect suggestion*. Irvington.

Farber, B.A. (2007). *Rock 'n' roll wisdom: What psychologically astute lyrics teach about life and love*. Praeger.

Farrelly, F., & Brandsma, J. (1974). *Provocative therapy*. Meta Publications.

Feldman, D.B., & Dreher, D.E. (2012). Can hope be changed in 90 minutes? Testing the efficacy of a single session goal-pursuit intervention for college students. *Journal of Happiness Studies, 13*(4), 745–759.

Feres, M., & Feres, M.F.N. (2023). Absence of evidence is not evidence of absence. *Journal of Applied Oral Science*.

Fisch, R. (1994). Basic elements in the brief therapies. In M.F. Hoyt (Ed.), *Constructive therapies* (pp. 126–139). Guilford Press.

Fisch, R., & Schlanger, K. (1999). *Brief therapy with intimidating cases: Changing the unchangeable*. Jossey-Bass.

Fisch, R., Weakland, J.H., & Segal, L. (1982). *The tactics of change: Doing therapy briefly*. Jossey-Bass.

Fleming, C. (2021). Single session family consultation with adults affected by eating disorders. In M.F. Hoyt, J. Young, & P. Rycroft (Eds.), *Single session thinking and practice in global, cultural, and familial contexts: Expanding applications* (pp. 305–314). Routledge.

Flemons, D., & Green, S. (2014). Quickies: Single session sex therapy. In M.F. Hoyt & M. Talmon (Eds.), *Capturing the moment: Single session therapy and walk-in services* (pp. 407–424). Crown House Publishing.

Follette, W.T., & Cummings, N.A. (1967). Psychiatric services and medical utilization in a prepaid health care setting. *Medical Care, 5,* 25–35.

Foster, R. (2009). *Personalismo* What's your approach? Medical Spanish blog. Retrieved online May 1, 2023.

Frances, A., & Clarkin, J.F. (1981). No treatment as the prescription of choice. *Archives of General Psychiatry, 38,* 542–545.

Frank, J.D. (1968). The role of hope in psychotherapy. *International Journal of Psychiatry, 6*, 383–395.

Frank, J.D. (1990). Foreword. In M. Talmon (Ed.), *Single-session therapy: Maximizing the effects of the first (and often only) therapeutic encounter* (pp. xi–xiii). Jossey-Bass.

Frank, J.D., & Frank, J.B. (1991). *Persuasion and healing: A comparative study of psychotherapy* (3rd ed.). Johns Hopkins University Press.

Frankl, V. (1963). *Man's search for meaning: An introduction to logotherapy*. Washington Square Press.

Freedman, J., & Combs, G. (1996). *Narrative therapy: The social construction of preferred realities*. Norton.

Freud, S. (1900). The analysis of dreams. In *The standard edition of the complete psychological works of Sigmund Freud* (Vols. 4 & 5). Hogarth Press, 1953.

Freud, S. (1917). Mourning and melancholia. In *The standard edition of the complete psychological works of Sigmund Freud* (Vol. 17). Hogarth Press, 1964.

Freud, S. (1937). Analysis terminable and interminable. In *Standard edition of the complete psychological works of Sigmund Freud* (Vol. 23, pp. 211–253). Hogarth Press, 1953–1974.

Friedman, S. (Ed.) (1993). *The new language of change: Constructive collaboration in psychotherapy*. Guilford Press.

Friedman, S. (1996). Couples therapy: Changing conversations. In H. Rosen & K.T. Kuehlwein (Eds.), *Constructing realities: Meaning-making perspectives for psychotherapists* (pp. 413–453). Jossey-Bass.

Friedman, S. (1997). *Time-effective psychotherapy: Maximizing outcomes in an era of minimized resources*. Allyn & Bacon.

Frykman, J. (2001, December 8). Nichole: An Erickson case, followed for 22 years. Workshop presented at the Eighth International Congress on Ericksonian Approaches to Hypnosis and Psychotherapy. Phoenix, AZ.

Fullen, C.T. (2020). The therapeutic alliance in a single session: A conversation analysis. *Journal of Systemic Therapies, 38*(4), 45–61.

Furman, B., & Ahola, T. (1992). *Solution talk: Hosting therapeutic conversations*. Norton.

Fuzzard, S. (2021). Embedding single session family consultation in a national youth mental health service: headspace. In M.F. Hoyt, J. Young, & P. Rycroft (Eds.), *Single session thinking and practice in global, cultural, and familial contexts: Expanding applications* (pp. 133–139). Routledge.

Fuzzard, S. (in press). Exploring SST / drop-ins around the world to increase access to timely mental health services and improve outcomes for young Australians. In F. Cannistrà & M.F. Hoyt (Eds.), *Single session therapies: Why and how one-at-a-time mindsets are effective*. Routledge, forthcoming.

Gawrysiak, M., Nicholas, C., & Hopko, D.R. (2009). Behavioral activation for moderately depressed university students: Randomized controlled trial. *Journal of Counseling Psychology, 56*(3), 468–476.

Geertz, C. (1973). *Local knowledge: Further essays in interpretive anthropology*. Basic Books.

George, E., Iveson, C., & Ratner, H. (1990). *Problem to solution: Brief therapy with individuals and families*. BT Press.

Gergen, K.J. (1993). Foreword. In S. Friedman (Ed.), *The new language of change: Constructive collaboration in psychotherapy* (pp. ix–xi). Guilford Press.

Gergen, K.J. (1998). Foreword. In M.F. Hoyt (Ed.), *The handbook of constructive therapies* (pp. xi–xv). Jossey-Bass.

Gergen, M.M., & Gergen, K.J. (Ed.) (1984). The social construction of narrative accounts. In *Historical social psychology* (pp. 173–189). Lawrence Erlbaum Publishers.

Gergen, K.J., & McNamee, S. (1991). *Therapy as social construction.* Sage.

Gibbons, J., & Plath, D. (2012). Single session work in hospitals. *Australian and New Zealand Journal of Family Therapy, 33*(1), 39–53.

Gilboa-Schectman, E., & Shafar, G. (2006). The sooner, the better: Temporal patterns in brief treatment of depression and their role in long-term outcome. *Psychotherapy Research, 16*(3), 374–384.

Gladwell, M. (2000). *The tipping point: How little things can make a big difference.* Brown, Little.

Goldfield, J.A. (1998). The master of faster. In M.F. Hoyt (Ed.), *The handbook of constructive therapies* (pp. 243–245). Jossey-Bass.

Goldfield, J.A., & Hoyt, M.F. (2022, September). Using progressive muscle relaxation to make embedded and embodied hypnotic suggestions *The Science of Psychotherapy, 10*(9), 32–44 (online).

Gordon, D., & Meyers-Anderson, M. (1981). *Phoenix: Therapeutic patterns of Milton H. Erickson.* Meta Publications.

Gould, G.S., & Watters, H.E. (2015). Are single-session smoking cessation groups a feasible option for rural Australia? – Outcomes from a pilot study. *Journal of Smoking Cessation, 10*(2), 135–140.

Goulding, M.M. (1990). Getting the important work done fast: Contract plus redecision. In J.K. Zeig & S.G. Gilligan (Eds.), *Brief therapy: Myths, methods, and metaphors* (pp. 303–317). Brunner/Mazel.

Goulding, M.M., & Goulding, R.L. (1979). *Changing lives through redecision therapy.* Brunner/Mazel.

Goulding, R.L., & Goulding, M.M. (1988). *Redecision therapy.* Videotape. International Transactional Analysis Association.

Green, S. (2014). Horse sense: Equine-assisted single session consultations. In M.F. Hoyt & M. Talmon (Eds.), *Capturing the moment: Single session therapy and walk-in services* (pp. 425–440). Crown House Publishing.

Greenleaf, E. (2013). Life is with people. In M.F. Hoyt (Ed.), *Therapist stories of inspiration, passion, and renewal: What's love to do with it?* (pp. 100–108). Routledge.

Grube, G.M.A. (1989). *Aristotle on poetry and style.* Hackett Publishing.

Gustafson, J.P. (1986). *The complex secret of brief psychotherapy.* Norton.

Gustafson, J.P. (2005). *Very brief psychotherapy.* Routledge.

Guthrie, B. (2018). Reflections on providing single-session therapy in post-disaster Haiti. In M.F. Hoyt et al. (Eds.), *Single session therapy by walk-in or appointment* (pp. 303–317). Routledge.

Haley, J. (1963). *Strategies of psychotherapy.* Grune & Stratton.

Haley, J. (1969). *The power tactics of Jesus Christ and other essays.* Avon.

Haley, J. (1973). *Uncommon therapy: The psychiatric techniques of Milton H. Erickson, M.D.* Norton.

Haley, J. (1977). *Problem-solving therapy: New strategies for effective family therapy.* Jossey-Bass.

Haley, J. (1982). The contribution to therapy of Milton H. Erickson, M.D. In J.K. Zeig (Ed.), *Ericksonian approaches to hypnosis and psychotherapy* (pp. 5–25). Brunner/Mazel.

Haley, J. (1984). *Ordeal therapy: Unusual ways to change behavior.* Jossey-Bass.

Haley, J. (1985). *Conversations with Milton H. Erickson, M.D.* (Vols. 1–3). Triangle Press.

Haley, J. (1989). *The first therapy session: How to interview clients and identify problems successfully.* Audiotape. Jossey-Bass.

Haley, J. (1990). Why not long-term therapy? In J.K. Zeig & S.G. Gilligan (Eds.), *Brief therapy: Myths, methods, and metaphors* (pp. 3–17). Brunner/Mazel.

Haley, J., & Richeport, M. (1993). *Milton H. Erikson, M.D.: Explorer in hypnosis and therapy.* Videotape/DVD. Brunner/Mazel.

Haley, J., & Richeport-Haley, M. (2003). *The art of strategic therapy.* Routledge.

Hammel, S. (2020). *Therapeutic interventions in three sentences: Reshaping Ericksonian hypnotherapy by talking to the brain and body.* Routledge. (Published originally in German in 2017.)

Hammerschlag, C. (1988). *The dancing healers: A doctor's journey of healing with Native Americans.* HarperCollins.

Hampson, R., O'Hanlon, J., Franklin, A., Pentony, M., Fridgant, L., & Heins, T. (1999). The place of single-session family consultation: Five years' experience in Canberra. *Australian and New Zealand Journal of Family Therapy, 20*(4), 195–200.

Hardy, K.V., & Bobes, T. (Eds.) (2016). *Culturally sensitive supervision and training: Diverse perspectives and practical suggestions.* Routledge.

Harper-Jaques, S. (2018). Supervision and the single-session therapist: Learnings from ten years of practice. In M.F. Hoyt et al., (Eds.), *Single session therapy by walk-in or appointment* (pp. 334–346). Routledge.

Harper-Jaques, S., & Foucault, D. (2014). Walk-in single-session therapy: Client satisfaction and clinical outcomes. *Journal of Systemic Therapies, 33*(3), 29–49.

Hartley, E., Moore, L., Knuckey, A., von Doussa, H., Painter, F., Story, K., Barrington, N., Young, J., & McIntosh, J. (2023). Walk-in together: A pilot study of a walk-in online family therapy intervention. *Australian and New Zealand Journal of Family Therapy, 44*(2), 127–144.

Henneberry, J. (2022). *A Foucauldian discourse analysis of the co-construction of client identity within a single-session therapy.* Unpublished doctoral dissertation. University of Ottawa.

Herman, J. (1992). *Trauma and recovery.* Basic Books.

Hill, R. (2018, December 12). *The art of client responsiveness in hypnotherapy and psychotherapy.* Short course at 13th International Congress on Ericksonian Approaches to Hypnosis and Psychotherapy. Phoenix, AZ.

Hill, R., & Rossi, E.L. (2017). *The practitioner's guide to mirroring hands: A client-responsive therapy that facilitates natural problem-solving and mind-body healing.* Crown House Publishing.

Hillman, J., & Ventura, M. (1992). *We've had a hundred years of psychotherapy – and the world's getting worse.* HarperCollins.

Hoagland, T. (2014). *Twenty poems that could save America, and other essays.* Graywolf Press.

Hoffman, L. (1990). Constructing realities: An art of lenses. *Family Process, 29*, 1–12. (Reprinted in *Exchanging voices: A collaborative approach to family therapy* (pp. 86–102). Karnac Books, 1993.)

Horowitz, M.J., Marmar, C., Krupnick, J., Wilner, N., Kaltreider, N., & Wallerstein, R. (1984). *Personality styles and brief psychotherapy.* Basic Books.

Hoyt, M.F. (1979) 'Patient' or 'client': What's in a name? *Psychotherapy: Theory, Research & Practice, 16*, 46–47. Reprinted in M.F. Hoyt, *Brief therapy and beyond* (pp. 1–2). Routledge, 2017.

Hoyt, M.F. (1985). 'Shrink' or 'expander': An issue in forming a therapeutic alliance. *Psychotherapy, 22*: 813–814. Reprinted in M.F. Hoyt, *Brief therapy and beyond* (pp. 3–5). Routledge, 2017.

Hoyt, M.F. (1990/2017). On time in brief therapy. In *Brief therapy and beyond: Stories, language, love, hope, and time* (pp. 6–32). Routledge. A slightly abbreviated version was originally published in R.A. Wells & V.J. Giannetti (Eds.), *Handbook of the brief psychotherapies*. Plenum, 1990.

Hoyt, M.F. (1991/1995). Teaching and learning short-term psychotherapy within an HMO. In C.S. Austad & W.H. Berman (Eds.), *Psychotherapy in managed health care: The optimal use of time and resources* (pp. 98–107). APA Books. (Reprinted in M.F. Hoyt, *Brief therapy and managed care* [pp. 63–68]. Jossey-Bass, 1995.)

Hoyt, M.F. (1994a). Introduction: Competency-based future-oriented therapy. In M.F. Hoyt (Ed.), *Constructive therapies* (pp. 1–10). Guilford Press.

Hoyt, M.F. (1994b). Single session solutions. In M.F. Hoyt (Ed.), *Constructive therapies* (pp. 140–159). Guilford Press.

Hoyt, M.F. (Ed.) (1994c). *Constructive therapies*. Guilford Press.

Hoyt, M.F. (1995a). *Brief therapy and managed care: Readings for contemporary practice*. Jossey-Bass.

Hoyt, M.F. (1995b). Therapist resistances to short-term dynamic psychotherapy. In M.F. Hoyt, *Brief therapy and managed care* (pp. 219–235). Jossey-Bass. (Work originally published in *Journal of the American Academy of Psychoanalysis*, 1985, *13*, 93–112.)

Hoyt, M.F. (1995c). Single-session solutions. In *Brief therapy and managed care* (pp. 141–162). Jossey-Bass. [A version was published earlier in M.F. Hoyt (Ed.), *Constructive Therapies* (pp. 140–159). New York: Guilford Press, 1994.]

Hoyt, M.F. (1995d). Contact, contract, change, encore: A conversation about redecision therapy with Bob Goulding. *Transactional Analysis Journal*, *25*(4), 300–311. (Reprinted in M.F. Hoyt, *Interviews with brief therapy experts* (pp. 121–143). Brunner-Routledge, 2001.)

Hoyt, M.F. (1996a). A golfer's guide to brief therapy (with footnotes for baseball fans). In M.F. Hoyt (Ed.), *Constructive therapies* (Vol. 2, pp. 306–318). Guilford Press. (Reprinted in M.F. Hoyt, *Brief therapy and beyond* (pp. 33–43). Routledge, 2017.)

Hoyt, M.F. (1996b). Haiku. In M.F. Hoyt (Ed.), *Constructive therapies* (Vol. 2, p. 375). Guilford Press.

Hoyt, M.F. (Ed.). (1996c). *Constructive therapies* (Vol. 2). Guilford Press.

Hoyt, M.F. (1997). Unmuddying the waters: A "common ground" conference. *Journal of Systemic Therapies*, *16*(3), 195–200. Reprinted in M.F. Hoyt, *Some stories are better than others* (pp. 195–200). Brunner/Mazel, 2000.

Hoyt, M.F. (1998a). Constructing therapeutic realities: A conversation with Paul Watzlawick. In M.F. Hoyt (Ed.), *Interviews with brief therapy experts* (pp. 144–157). Brunner/Routledge.

Hoyt, M.F. (Ed.) (1998b). *The handbook of constructive therapies*. Jossey-Bass.

Hoyt, M.F. (2000a). *Some stories are better than others: Doing what works in brief therapy and managed care*. Brunner/Mazel

Hoyt, M.F. (2000b). The last session in brief therapy: How and why to say "when." In *Some stories are better than others* (pp. 237–261). Brunner/Mazel.

Hoyt, M.F. (2000c). What can we learn from Milton Erickson's therapeutic failures? In *Some stories are better than others* (pp. 189–194). Brunner/Mazel.

Hoyt, M.F. (2000d). A single-session therapy retold: Evolving and restoried understandings. In *Some stories are better than others* (pp. 169–188). Brunner/Mazel. Reprinted in *Brief therapy and beyond* (pp. 134–152). Routledge, 2017.

Hoyt, M.F. (2001a) Solution building and language games: A conversation with Steve de Shazer (and some after words with Insoo Kim Berg). In M.F. Hoyt, *Interviews with brief therapy experts* (pp. 158–183). Brunner-Routledge. Work originally published in M.F. Hoyt (Ed.) (1996), *Constructive therapies* (Vol. 2, pp. 60–85). Guilford Press.

Hoyt, M.F. (2001b). On the importance of keeping it simple and taking the patient seriously: A conversation with Steve de Shazer and John Weakland. In M.F. Hoyt, *Interviews with brief therapy experts* (pp. 1–33). Brunner-Routledge. [Work originally published in M.F. Hoyt (Ed.), *Constructive therapies* (pp. 11–40). Guilford Press, 1994.]

Hoyt, M.F. (2001c). Connection: The doubled-edged gift of presence. *Journal of Clinical Psychology: In Session, 57*(8), 1–8. Reprinted and expanded in *Brief therapy and beyond* (pp. 179–188). Routledge, 2017.

Hoyt, M.F. (2001d). Direction and discovery: A conversation about power and politics in narrative therapy with Michael White and Jeff Zimmerman. In M.F. Hoyt, *Interviews with brief therapy experts* (pp. 265–293). Brunner-Routledge.

Hoyt, M.F. (2001e). Cognitive-behavioral treatment of posttraumatic stress disorder from a narrative constructivist perspective: A conversation with Donald Meichenbaum. In M.F. Hoyt, *Interviews with brief therapy experts* (pp. 97–120). Brunner-Routledge. [work originally published in M.F. Hoyt (Ed.), *Constructive therapies* (Vol. 2, 124–147). Guilford Press, 1996.]

Hoyt, M.F. (2002). How I embody a narrative constructive approach. *Journal of Constructivist Psychology, 15*, 279–289.

Hoyt, M.F. (2004). "The present is a gift": A clinical demonstration. In *The present is a gift: Mo' better stories from the world of brief therapy* (pp. 30–47). iUniverse.

Hoyt, M.F. (2008). Interview: Collaborative managed care. In N. Ruddy, D. Borresen, & W. Gunn (Eds.), *The collaborative psychotherapist: Creating reciprocal relationships with medical professionals* (pp. 195–203). APA Books.

Hoyt, M.F. (2009a). Solution-focused couple therapy. In M.F. Hoyt, *Brief psychotherapies: Principles and practices* (pp. 139–196). Zeig, Tucker, & Theisen.

Hoyt, M.F. (2009b). A few examples of my use of literature, music, and other arts in therapy. In *Brief psychotherapies: Principles and practices* (pp. 91–96). Zeig, Tucker, & Theisen.

Hoyt, M.F. (2009c). Brief psychotherapies: An introduction. In *Brief psychotherapies: Principles and practices* (pp. 1–76). Zeig, Tucker, & Theisen.

Hoyt, M.F. (2011) Foreword. In A. Slive & M. Bobele (Eds.), *When one hour is all you have: Effective therapy for walk-in clients* (pp. ix–xv). Zeig, Tucker, & Theisen.

Hoyt, M.F. (2012). Book review of S. Andreas, Transforming negative self-talk: Practical, effective exercises. *The Milton H. Erickson Foundation Newsletter, 32*(3), 19.

Hoyt, M.F. (2014). Psychology and my gallbladder: An insider's account of a single session therapy. In M.F. Hoyt & M. Talmon (Eds.), *Capturing the moment: Single session therapy and walk-in services* (pp. 53–72). Crown House Publishing.

Hoyt, M.F. (2015). Solution-focused couple therapy. In A.S. Gurman, J.L. Lebow, & D.K. Snyder (Eds.), *Clinical handbook of couple therapy* (5th ed., pp. 300–332). Guilford Press.

Hoyt, M.F. (2017). *Brief therapy and beyond: Stories, language, love, hope, and time.* Routledge.

Hoyt, M, F. (2018). Single-session therapy: Stories, structures, themes, cautions, and prospects. In M.F. Hoyt, M. Bobele, A. Slive, J. Young, & M. Talmon (Eds.), *Single-session therapy by walk-in or appointment: Administrative, clinical, and supervisory aspects of one- at-a-time services* (pp. 155–174). Routledge.

Hoyt, M.F. (2019a) Going "one-down." In M.F. Hoyt & M. Bobele (Eds.), *Creative therapy in challenging situations: Unusual interventions to help clients* (pp. 103–112). Routledge.

Hoyt, M.F. (2019b). Strategic therapies: Roots and branches. *Journal of Systemic Therapies, 38*(1), 30–43. A version reprinted as "Strategic Therapies: Past, Present, and Future" in V. Saladino (Ed.), *Le Strategie in psicoterapia: Ricerca e innovzione* (pp. 149–159). Bari, Italy: Cacucci Editore, 2021.

Hoyt, M.F. (2021). The hope and joy of SST. In M.F. Hoyt et al. (Eds.), *Single session thinking and practice in global, cultural, and familial contexts* (pp. 29–41). Routledge.

Hoyt, M.F. (2023, November 10). *The SST/OAAT mindset and using Single Session Thinking to teach an SST workshop.* Paper presented at 4th International SST Symposium. Rome, Italy.

Hoyt, M.F. (in press). Single session therapy. In R. Boland & M. Verduin (Eds.), *Kaplan & Sadock's comprehensive textbook of psychiatry* (11th ed.). Wolters Klower Publishers.

Hoyt, M.F. (in press b). The SST/OAAT mindset and using single session thinking to teach an SST workshop. In F. Cannistrà & M.F. Hoyt (Eds.), *Single session therapies: Why and how one-at-a-time mindsets are effective.* Routledge.

Hoyt, M.F., & Andreas, S. (2015). Humor in brief therapy. *Journal of Systemic Therapies, 34*(3), 14–25.

Hoyt, M.F., & Battino, R. (2021). When clients don't (and won't) change. *The Milton H. Erickson Foundation Newsletter, 41*(3), 8.

Hoyt, M.F., & Battino, R. (2022). On the importance of (occasionally) being unpredictable. *The Milton H. Erickson Foundation Newsletter, 42*(1), 12–13.

Hoyt, M.F., & Berg, I.K. (1998). Solution-focused couple therapy: Helping clients construct self- fulfilling prophecies. In M.F. Hoyt (Ed.), *The handbook of constructive therapies* (pp. 314–340). Jossey-Bass. Reprinted in M.F. Hoyt, *Some stories are better than others* (pp. 143–166). Brunner/Mazel, 2000.

Hoyt, M.F., Bobele, M., Slive, A., Young, J., & Talmon (Eds.) (2018a). *Single-session therapy by walk-in or appointment: Administrative, clinical, and supervisory aspects of one-at-a-time services.* Routledge. Published in Spanish as *Terapia de una sola session con o sin cita previa: Aspectos administrativos, clinicos y supervision de servicios de una sola vez.* Barcelona: Editorial Eleftheria, 2021. Published in German as *Wenn die Zeit knapp ist. Der Single-Session-Ansatz in Therapie und Beratung* [*When time is of the essence, the single session approach in therapy and counseling*] by Carl-Auer Verlag, Heidelburg, 2024.

Hoyt, M.F., Bobele, M., Slive, A., Young, J., & Talmon, M. (2018b). Single-session/one-at-a time walk-in therapy. In M.F. Hoyt, M. Bobele, J. Young, & M. Talmon (Eds.), *Single-session therapy by walk-in or appointment: Administrative, clinical, and supervisory aspects of one-at-a-time services* (pp. 3–24). Routledge.

Hoyt, M.F., & Cannistrà, F. (2023a). *Brief therapy conversations: Exploring efficient intervention in psychotherapy.* Routledge.

Hoyt, M.F., & Cannistrà, F. (2023b). Common errors in single session therapy. In *Brief therapy conversations: Exploring efficient intervention in psychotherapy* (pp. 157–169). Routledge. (An earlier version first appeared in *Journal of Systemic Therapies*, 2021, *40*(3), 29–41.)

Hoyt, M.F., & Dryden, W. (2018). Toward the future of single-session therapy: An interview. *Journal of Systemic Therapies, 37*(1), 79–89. Reprinted in W. Dryden, *Single-session therapy and its future: What SST leaders think* (pp. 31–45). New York: Routledge, 2021.

Hoyt, M.F., & Goulding, R.L. (1989). Resolution of a transference-countertransference impasse using Gestalt techniques in supervision. *Transactional Analysis Journal, 19*, 201–211. (Reprinted in M.F. Hoyt, *Brief therapy and managed care*, pp. 237–256. Jossey-Bass, 1995.)

Hoyt, M.F., Henley, M.D., & Collins, B.E. (1972). Studies in forced compliance: The confluence of choice and consequences on attitude change. *Journal of Personality and Social Psychology, 23*, 205–210.

Hoyt, M.F., & Janis, I.L. (1975). Increasing adherence to a stressful decision via a motivational balance-sheet procedure: A field experiment. *Journal of Personality and Social Psychology, 31*, 833–839. Reprinted in I.L. Janis, *Short-term counseling: Guidelines based on recent research*. Yale University Press, 1983.

Hoyt, M.F., & Miller, S.D. (2000). Stage-appropriate change-oriented brief therapy strategies. In M.F. Hoyt (Ed.), *Some stories are better than others* (pp. 207–235). Brunner/Mazel.

Hoyt, M.F., & Nylund, D. (1997). The joy of narrative: An exercise for learning from our internalized clients. *Journal of Systemic Therapies, 16*(4), 361–366. Adapted and reprinted in M.F. Hoyt (2000), *Some stories are better than others* (pp. 201–206). Brunner/Mazel.

Hoyt, M.F., & Ritterman, M. (2012). Brief therapy in a taxi. *The Milton H. Erickson Foundation Newsletter, 32*(2), 7.

Hoyt, M.F., & Rosenbaum, R. (2018). Some ways to end an SST. In M.F. Hoyt et al. (Eds.), *Single-session therapy by walk-in or appointment* (pp. 318–323). Routledge.

Hoyt, M.F., Rosenbaum, R., & Talmon, M. (1992). Planned single-session psychotherapy. In S.H. Budman, M.F. Hoyt, & S. Friedman (Eds.), *The first session in brief therapy* (pp. 59–86). Guilford Press.

Hoyt, M.F., & Talmon, M. (1990). Single-session therapy in action: A case example. In M. Talmon, *Single-session therapy: Maximizing the effect of the first (and often only) therapeutic encounter* (pp. 78–96). Jossey-Bass.

Hoyt, M.F., & Talmon, M. (Eds.) (2014). *Capturing the moment: Single session therapy and walk-in services*. Crown House Publishing.

Hoyt, M.F., Young, J., & Rycroft, P. (Eds.) (2021). *Single session thinking and practice in global, cultural, and familial contexts: Expanding applications*. Routledge.

Hubble, M.A., & O'Hanlon, W.H. (1992). Theory countertransference. *Dulwich Centre Newsletter, 1*, 25–30.

Hudson, P.O., & O'Hanlon, W.H. (1992). *Rewriting love stories: Brief marital therapy*. Norton.

Hurn, R. (2005). Single-session therapy: Planned success or unplanned failure? *Counselling Psychology Review, 20*(4), 33–40.

Hymmen, P., Stalker, C., & Cait, C.-A. (2013). The case for single-session therapy: Does the empirical evidence support the increased prevalence of this service delivery model? *Journal of Mental Health, 22*(1), 60–71.

Iveson, C. (1990). *Whose life? Community care of older people and their families*. Brief Therapy Press.

Iveson, C. (2019). However great the question, it's the answer that makes a difference. In M.F. Hoyt & M. Bobele (Eds.), *Creative therapy in challenging situations: Unusual interventions to help clients* (pp. 121–133). Routledge.

Iveson, C., George, E., & Ratner, H. (2012). *Brief coaching: A solution-focused approach*. Routledge.

Iveson, C., George, E., & Ratner, H. (2014). Love is all around: A single session solution-focused therapy. In M.F. Hoyt & M. Talmon (Eds.), *Capturing the moment: Single session therapy and walk-in services* (pp. 325–348). Crown House Publishing.

Jacobson, G. (1968). The briefest psychiatric encounter: Acute effects of evaluation. *Archives of General Psychiatry, 18*, 718–724.

Jacobson, N.S., Martell C.R., & Dimidjian, S. (2001). Behavioral activation treatment for depression: Returning to contextual roots. *Clinical Psychology: Science and Practice, 8*(3), 255–270.

James, C. (2014). *Poetry notebook: Reflections on the intensity of language.* Liveright/Norton.

James, W. (1890). *The principles of psychology* (Vol. 2). Henry Holt & Company.

Jerry, P.A. (1994). *Winnicott's therapeutic consultation and the adolescent client. Crisis Intervention and Time-Limited Treatment, 1*, 61–72.

Jevne, R., Zingle, H., Ryan, D., McDougall, C., & Moretmore, E. (1995). Single-session therapy for teachers with a health disabling condition. *Employee Counselling Today, 7*(1), 5–11.

Jones, C. (1985). Strategic interventions within a no-treatment frame. *Family Process, 24*, 583–595.

Jones, J.D. (2005). A comparison of songwriting and lyric analysis techniques to evoke emotional change in a single session with people who are chemically dependent. *Journal of Music Therapy, 43*(2), 94–110.

Jones, M.P., Kadlubek, R.M, & Marks, M.J. (2006). Single-session treatment: A counseling paradigm for school psychology. *The School Psychologist, 60*, 123–115.

Joseph, J. (2023, November 10). A comprehensive biometric analysis of Single Session Therapy: Insights and implications. Paper presented at 4th International Symposium on Single Session Therapy, Rome.

Josling, L., & Cait, C.-A. (2018). The walk-in counseling model: Research and advocacy. In M.F. Hoyt et al. (Eds.), *Single-session therapy by walk-in or appointment* (pp. 91–103). Routledge.

Kachor, M., & Brothwell, J. (2020). Improving youth mental health services access using a single-session therapy approach. *Journal of Systemic Therapies, 39*(3), 46–55.

Kahneman, D. (2011). *Thinking, fast and slow.* Farrar, Straus and Giroux.

Karrass, C.L. (1992). *The negotiating game* (rev. ed.). HarperCollins.

Kashdan, T.B., Adams, L., Read, J., & Hawk, Jr., L. (2012). Can a one-hour session of exposure treatment modulate startle response and reduce spider fears? *Psychiatric Research, 196*, 79–82.

Kazantzakis, N. (1965). *Report to Greco.* Simon & Schuster. (Work originally published in 1957 in Greek.)

Keeney, H., & Keeney, B. (2013). *Creative therapeutic technique: Skills for the art of bringing forth change.* Zeig, Tucker, & Theisen.

Keeney, H., & Keeney, B. (2014). Deconstructing therapy: Case study of a single session crisis intervention. In M.F. Hoyt & M. Talmon (Eds.), *Capturing the moment: Single session therapy and walk-in services* (pp. 441–462). Crown House Publishing.

Keeney, H., & Keeney, B. (2019). 120 centimeters from sainthood. In M.F. Hoyt & M. Bobele (Eds.), *Creative therapy in challenging situations: Unusual interventions to help clients* (pp. 134–144). Routledge.

Keith, D.V. (2015). *Continuing the experiential approach of Carl Whitaker: Process, practice, and magic.* Zeig, Tucker, & Theisen.

Keith, D.V. (2019). Random effects of ambiguity along the pathway toward health. In M.F. Hoyt & M. Bobele (Eds.), *Creative therapy in challenging situations: Unusual interventions to help clients* (pp. 144–155). Routledge.

Kellner, R., Neidhardt, J., Krakow, B., & Pathak, D. (1992). Changes in chronic nightmares after one session of desensitization or rehearsal instruction. *American Journal of Psychiatry, 149*, 659–663.

Kim, J., Ryu, N., & Chibanda, D. (2023). Effectiveness of single-session therapy for adult common mental disorders: A systematic review. *BMC Psychology, 11*(373). Open access.

Kirschman, E., Kamena, M., & Fay, J. (2014). *Counseling cops: What clinicians need to know.* Guilford Press.

Koegler, R.R., & Cannon, J.A. (1966). Treatment for the many. *International Psychiatry Clinics, 3*(4), 93–105.

Kornfield, J. (1993). *A path with heart: A guide through the perils and promises of spiritual life.* Bantam.

Korngold, M. (2013). Herman's wager. In M.F. Hoyt (Ed.), *Therapist stories of inspiration, passion, and renewal: What's love got to do with it?* (pp. 163–174). Routledge.

Kottler, J. (2019). When impatience gets the best of me. In M.F. Hoyt & M. Bobele (Eds.), *Creative therapy in challenging situations: Unusual interventions to help clients* (pp. 156–162). Routledge.

Kuehn, J.L. (1965). Encounter at Leyden: Gustav Mahler consults Sigmund Freud. *Psychoanalytic Review, 52*, 345–364.

Kutz, I., Resnick, V., & Dekel, R. (2008). The effect of single-session modified EMDR on acute stress syndromes. *Journal of EMDR Practice and Research, 2*(3), 190–200.

Lamprecht, H., Laydon, C., McQuillan, C., Wiseman, S., Williams, L., Gash, A., & Reilly, J. (2007). Single-session solution-focused brief therapy and self-harm: A pilot study. *Journal of Psychiatric and Mental Health Nursing, 14*, 601–602.

Lamsal, R., Stalker, C.A., Cait, C.-A., Riemer, M., & Horton, S. (2018) Cost-effectiveness analysis of single-session walk-in counselling. *Journal of Mental Health, 27*(6), 560–566. https://doi.org/10.1080/09638237.2017.1340619

Lankton, S.R. (2001, December). *The basic footprint of Erickson's work.* Keynote address at Eighth International Congress on Ericksonian Approaches to Hypnosis and Psychotherapy. Phoenix, AZ.

Lazarus, A.A. (1971). *Behavior therapy and beyond.* McGraw-Hill.

Lazarus, A.A. (1993). Tailoring the therapeutic relationship, or being an authentic chameleon. *Psychotherapy: Theory, Research, & Practice, 30*(3), 404–407.

Le Gros, J., Wyder, M., & Brunelli, V. (2018). Single session work: Implementing brief intervention as routine practice in an acute care mental health assessment service. *Australasian Psychiatry, 27*(1), 21–24.

Leibenluft, E., Tasman, A., & Green, S.A. (Eds.) (1993). *Less time to do more: Psychotherapy on the short-term inpatient unit.* American Psychiatric Press.

LeShan, L. (1982). *The gardener and the mechanic: Making the most of the holistic revolution in medicine.* Holt.

Leslie, P.J. (2019). *The art of creating a magical session: Key elements for transformative psychotherapy.* Routledge.

Levin, S.B., Gil-Wilkerson, A., & Rapini De Yatim, S. (2018). Single-session walk-ins as a collaborative learning community at the Houston Galveston Institute. In M.F. Hoyt et al. (Eds.), *Single-session therapy by walk-in or appointment* (pp. 251–259). Routledge.

Lewin, K.K. (1970). *Brief psychotherapy: Brief encounters.* Warren H. Green Publishers.

Lewis, C.S (1956). *Surprised by joy.* Harcourt Brace Jovanovich.

Littrell, J.M., Malia, J.A., & Vanderwood, M. (1992). Single-session brief counseling in a high school. *Journal of Counseling and Development, 73* (March/April), 451–458.

Loriedo, C., & Vella, G. (1992). *Paradox and the family system.* Brunner/Mazel.

Lutz, A.B. (2014). *Learning solution-focused therapy: An illustrated guide.* American Psychiatric Press.

Madigan. S. (2019). *Narrative therapy.* APA Books.

Mahrer, A.R., & Roberge, M. (1993). Single-session experiential therapy with any person whatsoever. In R.A. Wells & V.J. Giannetti (Eds.), *Casebook of the brief psychotherapies* (pp. 179–196). Plenum Press.

Malan, D.H. (1976a). *The frontier of brief psychotherapy.* Plenum.

Malan, D.H. (1976b). *Toward the validation of dynamic psychotherapy.* Plenum.

Malan, D.H., Bacal, H.A., Heath, E.S., & Balfour, F.H.G. (1968). A study of psychodynamic changes in untreated neurotic patients: Improvements that are questionable on dynamic criteria. *British Journal of Psychiatry, 114*, 525–551.

Malan, D.H., Health, E.S., Bacal, H.A., & Balfour, F.H. (1975). Psychodynamic changes in untreated neurotic patients, II: Apparently genuine improvements. *Archives of General Psychiatry, 32*(1), 110–126.

Mandlik, G.V., Siopis, G., Nguyen, B., Ding, D., Edwards, K.M. (2023, October 11). Effect of a single session of yoga and meditation on stress reactivity: A systematic review. *Stress and Health.* Open access. https://doi.org/10.1002/smi.3324

Mann, J. (1973). *Time-limited psychotherapy.* Harvard University Press.

Marrow, A.J. (1977). *The practical theorist: The life and work of Kurt Lewin.* Teachers College Press.

Matthews, K.M. (2018). The integration of emotion-focused therapy within single-session therapy. *Journal of Systemic Therapies, 37*(4), 15–28.

May, R., Angel, E., & Ellenberger, H.F. (Eds.) (1958). *Existence: A new dimension in psychiatry and psychology.* Basic Books.

McCambridge, J., & Strong, J. (2004). The efficacy of single-session motivational interviewing in reducing drug consumption and perceptions of drug-related risk and harm among young people: Results from a multi-site cluster randomized trial. *Addiction, 99*(1), 39–52.

McDonald, J., Hickey, P., & Wyder, M. (2021). Implementing single session thinking in a public mental health setting in Queensland: Part II – Adapting and integrating single session therapy into an acute care setting. In M.F. Hoyt, J. Young, & P. Rycroft (Eds.), *Single session thinking and practice in global, cultural, and familial contexts* (pp. 110–116). Routledge.

McElheran, N. (2021). The story of the Eastside Family Centre: 30 years of walk-in single session therapy. In M.F. Hoyt, J. Young, & P. Rycroft (Eds.), *Single session thinking and practice in global, cultural, and familial contexts* (pp. 125–132). Routledge.

McElheran. N. (in press). Walk-in single sessions, then and now: The Eastside Community Mental Health Service. In F. Cannistrà & M.F. Hoyt (Eds.), *Single session therapies: Why and how one-at-a-time mindsets are effective.* Routledge, forthcoming.

McGoldrick, M., Giordano, J., & Garcia-Preto, N. (Eds.) (2005). *Ethnicity and family therapy* (3rd ed.). Guilford Press.

McKergow, M. (2016). SFBT 2.0: The next generation of solution-focused brief therapy has already arrived. *Journal of Solution Focused Practices, 2*(2), Article 3. Available at: https://digitalscholarship.unlv.edu/journalsfp/vol2/iss2/3

McKergow, M. (2021). *The next generation of solution focused practice: Stretching the world for new opportunities and progress*. Routledge.

McNamee, S., & Gergen, K.J. (Eds.). (1992) *Therapy as social construction*. Sage.

McNeel, J. (1976). The parent interview. *Transactional Analysis Journal, 6*, 61–68.

McNeilly, R. (1994). Solution-oriented counseling: A 20-minute format for medical practice. *Australian Family Physician, 23*, 228–230.

Mead, G.H. (1934). *Mind, self, and society*. University of Chicago Press.

Meichenbaum, D.H. (1985). *Stress inoculation training: A clinical guidebook*. Pergamon.

Meichenbaum, D.H. (2012). *Roadmap to resilience: A guide for military, trauma victims and their families*. Melissa Institute Press.

Meichenbaum, D.H. (2023). *Core tasks of psychotherapy: The art of questioning, motivational interviewing, single session therapy and psycho-educational procedures*. Melissa Institute Press.

Miller, J.K. (2008). Walk-in single-session team therapy: A study of client satisfaction. *Journal of Systemic Therapies, 27*(3), 78–94.

Miller, J.K. (2011). Single-session intervention in the wake of hurricane Katrina: Strategies for disaster mental health counseling. In A. Slive & M. Bobele (Eds.), *When one hour is all you have: Effective therapy for walk-in clients* (pp. 185–202). Zeig, Tucker, & Theisen.

Miller, J.K. (2014). Single session therapy in China. In M.F. Hoyt & M. Talmon (Eds.), *Capturing the moment: Single session therapy and walk-in services* (pp. 195–214). Crown House Publishing.

Miller, J.K., Platt, J.J., & Conroy, K.M. (2018). Single-session therapy in the majority world: Addressing the challenge of service delivery in Cambodia and its implications for other global contexts. In M.F. Hoyt et al. (Eds.), *Single-session therapy by walk-in or appointment* (pp. 116–134). Routledge.

Miller, J.K., & Slive, A. (2004). Breaking down the barriers to clinical service delivery: Walk-in family therapy. *Journal of Marital and Family Therapy, 30*, 95–105.

Miller, J.K., Xing, D., Yaorui, H., & Yilin, X. (2021). Single session team family therapy (SSTFT) in China: A seven-step protocol for adapting Western methods in Eastern contexts. In M.F. Hoyt, J. Young, & P. Rycroft (Eds.), *Single session thinking and practice in global, cultural, and familial contexts* (pp. 245–254). Routledge.

Miller, S.D. (1992). The symptoms of solution. *Journal of Strategic and Systemic Therapies, 11*, 1–11.

Miller, W.R. (2000). Rediscovering fire: Small interventions, large effects. *Psychology of Addictive Behaviors, 14*(1), 6–18.

Miller, W.R., & C'de Baca, J. (2001). *Quantum change: When epiphanies and sudden insights transform ordinary lives*. Guilford Press.

Miller, W.R., & Rollnick, S. (1991). *Motivational interviewing: Preparing people to change addictive behavior*. Guilford Press.

Minuchin, S. (1974). *Families and family therapy*. Harvard University Press.

Minuchin, S., & Nichols, M.P. (1998). *Family healing: Strategies for hope and understanding*. Free Press.

Mitchell, C.L., & Dorian, E.H. (Eds.). *Police psychology and its growing impact on modern law enforcement*. IGI Global.

Monk, G., Winslade, J., Crocket, K., & Epston, D. (Eds.) (1996). *Narrative therapy in practice: The archeology of hope*. Jossey-Bass.

Moore, L., Knucky, A., Barrington, N., Tsorlinis, K., George, E., Story, K., Hartley, E., McIntosh, J., & Young, J. (in press). Walk-in together: Online therapy for families, when and where they want it. In A. Slive & M. Bobele (Eds.), *Open access/one-at-a-time single session psychotherapy*. Routledge, forthcoming. Routledge.

Morrill, R.G. (1978). The future for mental health in primary care programs. *American Journal of Psychiatry, 135*, 1351–1355.

Morson, G.S. (1994). *Narrative and freedom: The shadows of time*. Yale University Press.

Mulligan, J., Olivieri, H., Young, K., Lin, J., & Anthony, S.J. (2022). Single session therapy in pediatric healthcare: The value of adopting a strengths-based approach for families living with neurological disorders. *Child and Adolescent Psychiatry and Mental Health, 16*, 59.

Mumford, E., Schlesinger, H., Glass, G.V., Patrick, C., & Cuerdon, B.A. (1984). A new look at evidence about reduced cost of medical utilization following mental health treatment. *American Journal of Psychiatry, 141*, 1145–1158.

Murphy, J.J. (2023). *Solution-focused counseling in schools* (4th ed.). American Counseling Association.

Murphy, J.J. (2024). *Solution-focused therapy*. APA Books.

Nardone, G. (in press). Strategic dialogue and hypnotherapy without trance. In F. Cannistrà & M.F. Hoyt (Eds.), *Single session therapies: Why and how one-at-a-time mindsets are effective*. Routledge, forthcoming.

Nardone, G., & Portelli, C. (2005). *Knowing through changing: The evolution of brief strategic therapy*. Crown House Publishing.

Nardone, G., & Salvini, A. (2018). *The strategic dialogue: Rendering the diagnostic interview a real therapeutic intervention*. Routledge.

Nardone, G., & Watzlawick, P. (1990). *The art of change: Strategic therapy and hypnotherapy without trance*. Jossey-Bass.

Nardone, G., & Watzlawick, P. (2005). *Brief strategic therapy: Philosophy, techniques, and research*. Jason Aronson Publishers.

Neimeyer, R.A. (1998). Cognitive therapy and the narrative trend: A bridge too far? *Journal of Cognitive Psychotherapy, 12*, 57–65.

Norcross, J.C. (Ed.). (2011). *Psychotherapy relationships that work: Therapist contributions and responsiveness to patients* (2nd ed.). Oxford University Press.

Nùñez, R., & Abia, J. (2021). Single session Ericksonian strategic hypnotherapy for disasters in Mexico. In M.F. Hoyt, J. Young, & P. Rycroft (Eds.), *Single session thinking and practice in global, cultural, and familial contexts* (pp. 255–263). Routledge.

Nuthall, A., & Townend, M. (2007). CBT-based early intervention to prevent panic disorder: A pilot study. *Behavioral and Cognitive Psychotherapy, 35*(1), 15–30.

Nylund, D., & Corsiglia, V. (1993). Internalized other questioning with men who are violent. In M.F. Hoyt (Ed.), *The handbook of constructive therapies* (pp. 401–413). Jossey-Bass.

Nylund, D., & Corsiglia, V. (1994). Becoming solution-focused/forced in brief therapy: Remembering something important we already knew. *Journal of Systemic Therapies, 13*, 5–12.

O'Hanlon, B., & Rottem, N. (2021). Single session family consultation (SSFC). In M.F. Hoyt, J. Young, & P. Rycroft (Eds.), *Single session thinking and practice in global, cultural, and familial contexts* (pp. 66–76). Routledge.

O'Hanlon, W.H. (1990). A grand unified theory for brief therapy: Putting problems in context. In J.K. Zeig & S.G. Gilligan (Eds.), *Brief therapy: Myths, methods, and metaphors* (pp. 78–89). Brunner/Mazel.

O'Hanlon, W.H. (1996). Tranceplants. In M.F. Hoyt (Ed.), *Constructive therapies* (Vol. 2, p. 369). Guilford Press.

O'Hanlon, W.H. (1999). *Do one thing different: And other uncommonly sensible solutions to life's persistent problems*. William Morrow.

O'Hanlon, W.H. (2003). *A guide to inclusive therapy: 26 methods of respectful, resistance-dissolving therapy*. Norton.

O'Hanlon, W.H., & Hexum, A.L. (1990). *An uncommon casebook: The complete clinical work of Milton H. Erickson, M.D.* Norton.

O'Hanlon, W.H., & Weiner-Davis, M. (1989). *In search of solutions: A new direction in psychotherapy*. Norton.

O'Hanlon, W.H., & Wilk, J. (1987). *Shifting contexts: The generation of effective psychotherapy*. Guilford Press.

Ollendick, T.H., & Davis, T.E. (2013). One-session treatment for specific phobias: A review of Öst's single-session exposure with children and adolescents. *Cognitive and Behavior Therapy, 42*(4), 275–83. https://doi.org/10.1080/16506073.2013.773062.

Ollendick, T.H., Öst, L.G., Reuterskiold, L., Costa, N., Cederlund, R., Sirbu, C., & Davis, T.E. (2009). One-session treatment of specific phobias in youth: A randomized clinical trial in the United States and Sweden. *Journal of Consulting and Clinical Psychology, 77*(3), 504–516.

O'Loughlin, K. (2021). Single session therapy for people with a new HIV diagnosis: Achieving a positive result. In M.F. Hoyt, J. Young, & P. Rycroft (Eds.), *Single session thinking and practice in global, cultural, and familial contexts: Expanding applications* (pp. 202–209). Routledge.

O'Neill I. (2017) What's in a name? Clients' experiences of single session therapy. *Journal of Family Therapy, 39*(1), 63–79.

Oremland, J.D. (1976). A curious resolution of a hysterical symptom. *International Review of Psycho-Analysis, 3*, 473–477.

Orne, M.T. (1969). Demand characteristics and the concept of quasi-controls. In R. Rosenthal & R.L. Rosnow (Eds.), *Artifacts in behavioral research* (pp. 143–179). Academic Press.

Öst, L.-G., Svensson, L., Hellström, K., & Lindwall, R. (2001). One-session treatment of specific phobias in youths: A randomized clinical trial. *Journal of Consulting and Clinical Clinical Psychology, 69*, 814–824.

Ozaki, N. (2017). *A conversation analysis of therapist-client interactional patterns in single session therapy: A researcher's interpretation*. Unpublished doctoral dissertation. Nova Southeastern University.

Paglia, C. (1992). *Sex, art, and American culture*. Vintage.

Palazzoli, M.S., Cecchin, G., Prata, G., & Boscolo, L. (1978). *Paradox and counterparadox: A new model in the therapy of the family in schizophrenic transaction*. Jason Aronson Publisher.

Paré, D. (2008). Crossing the divide: The therapeutic use of internalized other interviewing. *Journal of Clinical Activities, Assignments & Handouts, 1*(4), 21–28.

Paul, K.E., & van Ommeren, M. (2013). A primer on single session therapy and its potential application in humanitarian situations. *Intervention: Journal of Mental Health and Psychological Support in Conflict-Affected Areas, 11*(1), 8–23.

Paz, O. (1963). The endless instant/¿No hay salida? In D. Levertov (Trans.), *Early poems 1935–1955* (pp. 124–125). New Directions.

Peet, B. (1972). *The ant and the elephant*. Houghton Mifflin.

Pelletier, K.R. (1977). *Mind as healer, mind as slayer*. Delta.

Perdomo, C. (2017). Undocumented and deportable: Re-authoring trauma within the context of immigration in a narrative informed single session. *Journal of Systemic Therapies, 36*(4), 3–15.

Perkins, R. (2006). The effectiveness of one session of therapy using a single-session therapy approach for children and adolescents with mental health problems. *Psychology and Psychotherapy: Theory, Research and Practice, 79*, 215–227.

Perkins, R., & Scarlett, G. (2008). The effectiveness of single session therapy in child and adolescent mental health. Part 2: An 18-month follow-up study. *Psychology and Psychotherapy: Theory, Research and Practice, 81*, 143–156.

Perls, F. (1969). *Gestalt therapy verbatim*. Real People Press.

Phillips, P. (2002). Shoulder to shoulder: A single session success story. *Journal of College Student Psychotherapy, 16*(3/4), 225–237.

Piccirilli, F., & Ermini, L. (2023). The single-session therapy mindset. In F. Cannistrà & F. Piccirilli (Eds.), *Single-session therapy: Principles and practice* (pp. 51–66). Giunti. (Published in Italian in 2018.)

Pietrabissa, G. (in press). Single-session therapy: Exploring research evidence and frontiers. In F. Cannistrà & M.F. Hoyt (Eds.), *Single session therapies: Why and how one-at-a-time mindsets are effective*. Routledge, forthcoming.

Pirandello, L. (1921). *Six characters in search of an author*. (E. Bentley, Trans.). Signet Classics, 1998.

Pitt, T., Thomas, O., Lindsay, P., Hanton, S., & Bawden, M. (2015). Doing sports psychology briefly? A critical review of single session therapeutic approaches and their relevance to sport psychology. *International Review of Sport and Exercise Psychology, 8*(1), 125–155.

Platt, J.J., & Mondellini, D. (2014). Single session walk-in therapy for street robbery victims in Mexico City. In M.F. Hoyt & M. Talmon (Eds.), *Capturing the moment* (pp. 215–231). Crown House Publishing.

Porter, S., & Pitt, T. (2023, November 10). An expert opinion on the application of the Single Session mindset. Paper presented at 4th International Symposium on Single Session Therapy, Rome.

Preston, J., Varzos, N., & Liebert, D. (1995). *Every session counts: Making the most of your brief therapy*. Impact Publishers.

Prochaska, J.O. (1999). How do people change and how can we change to help many more people? In M.A. Hubble, B.L. Duncan, & S.D. Miller (Eds.), *The heart and soul of change: What works in therapy*. APA Books.

Quick, E.K. (1996). *Doing what works in brief therapy: A strategic solution focused approach*. Academic Press.

Rabba, A.S. (2021). Strengthening family resilience using a single session mindset following a child's diagnosis of autism. In M.F. Hoyt, J. Young, & P. Rycroft (Eds.), *Single session thinking and practice in global, cultural, and familial contexts: Expanding applications* (pp. 182–191). Routledge.

Ratner, H., George, E., & Iveson, C. (2012). *Solution focused brief therapy: 100 key points and techniques*. Routledge.

Ratner, H., & Yusef, D. (2015). *Brief coaching with children and young people*. Routledge.

Rausch, S. M., Gramling, S. E., & Auerbach, S. M. (2006). Effects of a single session of large-group meditation and progressive muscle relaxation training on stress reduction, reactivity, and recovery. *International Journal of Stress Management, 13*(3), 273–290.

Read, A., Mazzuccelli, T.G., & Kane, R.T. (2016). A preliminary evaluation of a single session behavioral activation intervention to improve well-being and prevent depression in carers. *Clinical Psychologist, 20*(1), 36–45.

Renkin, C., Alexander, K., & Wyder, M. (2021). Implementing single session thinking in public mental health settings in Queensland: Part I – Introducing single session family consultations into adult inpatient and community care. In M.F. Hoyt, J. Young, & P. Rycroft (Eds.), *Single session thinking and practice in global, cultural, and familial contexts: Expanding applications* (pp. 101–109). Routledge.

Reuss, N.H. (1997). The nightmare question. *Journal of Family Psychotherapy, 8*(4), 71–76.

Ritterman, M. (1985). Family context, symptom induction, and therapeutic counterinduction: Breaking the spell of a dysfunctional rapport. In J.K. Zeig (Ed.), *Ericksonian hypnotherapy: Clinical applications* (pp. 49–70). Brunner/Mazel.

Ritterman, M. (2005). *Using hypnosis in family therapy* (2nd ed.). Zeig, Tucker, & Theisen.

Ritterman, M. (2009). *The tao of a woman: 100 ways to turn.* Skipping Stones Editions.

Ritterman, M. (2014). One session therapy: Fast new stance using the slo-mo three-minute trance. In M.F. Hoyt & M. Talmon (Eds.), *Capturing the moment: Single session therapy and walk-in services* (pp. 373–392). Crown House Publishing.

Ritterman, M. (2019). The single stroke: What makes "zingers" zing? In M.F. Hoyt & M. Bobele (Eds.), *Creative therapy in challenging situations: Unusual interventions to help clients* (pp. 163–171). Routledge.

Robinson, A.M., Harvey, G., McDonald, M., & Honegger, T. (2021). Introducing single session therapy at a university counseling center. In M.F. Hoyt, J. Young, & P. Rycroft (Eds.), *Single session thinking and practice in global, cultural, and familial contexts* (pp. 143–152). Routledge.

Robinson, P.J., & Reiter, J.T. (2016). *Behavioral consultation in primary care: A guide to integrating services* (2nd ed.). Springer.

Robinson, P.J., Strosahl, K.D., & Gustavsson, T. (2012). *Brief interventions for radical change: Principles and practice of focused Acceptance and Commitment Therapy.* New Harbinger Publications.

Rockwell, W.J.K., & Pinkerton, R.S. (1982). Single-session psychotherapy. *American Journal of Psychotherapy, 36*, 32–40.

Rodda, S.N., Lubman, D.I., Cheetham, A., Dowling, N.A., & Jackson, A.C. (2015). Single session web-based counseling: A thematic analysis of content from the perspective of the client. *British Journal of Guidance and Counselling, 43*(1), 117–130.

Rodda, S.N., Lubman, D.I., Jackson, A.C., & Dowling, N.A. (2017). Improved outcomes following a single session web-based intervention for problem gambling. *Journal of Gambling Studies, 33*(1), 283–299.

Rodriguez, I.J. (2018). *Terapia breve sin cita:* Collaboration with a marginalized community in Mexico City. In M.F. Hoyt et al. (Eds.), *Single-session therapy by walk-in or appointment* (pp. 291–302). Routledge.

Rosenbaum, R. (1982). Paradox as epistemological jump. *Family Process, 21*(1), 85–90.

Rosenbaum, R. (1990). Strategic therapy. In R.A. Wells & V.J. Giannetti (Eds.), *Handbook of the brief psychotherapies* (pp. 351–403). New York: Plenum Press.

Rosenbaum, R. (1993). Heavy ideals: Strategic single-session hypnotherapy. In R.A. Wells & V.J. Giannetti (Eds.), *Casebook of the brief psychotherapies* (pp. 109–128). Plenum Press.

Rosenbaum, R. (1999). *Zen and the heart of psychotherapy.* Brunner-Routledge.

Rosenbaum, R. (2008). Psychotherapy is not short or long. *Monitor on Psychology, 39*(7), 4, 8.

Rosenbaum, R. (2013). *Walking the way: 81 Zen encounters with the Tao Te Ching*. Wisdom Publications.

Rosenbaum, R. (2014). The time of your life. In M.F. Hoyt & M. Talmon (Eds.), *Capturing the moment: Single session therapy and walk-in services* (pp. 41–52). Crown House Publishing.

Rosenbaum, R. (2021). Gradually and suddenly: What Zen teaches us about change in SST. In M.F. Hoyt, J. Young, & P. Rycroft (Eds.), *Single session thinking and practice in global, cultural, and familial contexts* (pp. 89–97). Routledge.

Rosenbaum, R. (2022). *That is not your mind! Zen reflections on the Surangama Sutra*. Shambhala Publications.

Rosenbaum, R. (in press). Beyond is and is-not. In F. Cannistrà & M.F. Hoyt (Eds.), *Single session therapies: Why and how one-at-a-time mindsets are effective*. Routledge, forthcoming.

Rosenbaum, R., & Bohart, A.C. (2007). Psychotherapy: The art of experience. In S. Krippner, M. Bova, & L. Grat (Eds.), *Healing stories: The use of narrative in counseling and psychotherapy* (pp. 295–324). Puente Press.

Rosenbaum, R., Hoyt, M.F., & Talmon, M. (1990). The challenge of single-session therapies: Creating pivotal moments. In R.A. Wells & V.J. Giannetti (Eds.), *Handbook of the brief psychotherapies* (pp. 165–189). Plenum. Reprinted in M.F. Hoyt, *Brief therapy and managed care: Readings for contemporary practice* (pp. 105–139). Jossey-Bass, 1995.

Rosenberg, T., & McDaniel, S.H. (2014). Single session medical family therapy and the patient- centered medical home. In M.F. Hoyt & M. Talmon (Eds.), *Capturing the moment: Single session therapy and walk-in services* (pp. 349–362). Crown House Publishing.

Rossi, E.L. (1973). Psychological shocks and creative moments in psychotherapy. *American Journal of Clinical Hypnosis, 16*, 9–22.

Rossi, E.L. (1996). *The symptom path to enlightenment*. Palisades Gateway Publishing.

Rossi, E.L., & Cheek, D.L. (1988). *Mind-body therapy: Methods of ideodynamic healing in hypnosis*. Norton.

Rossi, K., & Rossi, E.L. (2014). Opening the heart and mind with single session psychotherapy and therapeutic hypnosis: A final meeting with Milton H. Erickson, M.D. – Part I. In M.F. Hoyt & M. Talmon (Eds.), *Capturing the moment: Single session therapy and walk-in services* (pp. 233–253). Crown House Publishing.

Rycroft, P. (2018). Capturing the moment in supervision. In M.F. Hoyt et al. (Eds.), *Single-session therapy by walk-in or appointment* (pp. 347–365). Routledge.

Rycroft, P. (in press). Finding the beauty in every encounter: The aesthetics of a single session. In F. Cannistrà & M.F. Hoyt (Eds.), *Single session therapies: Why and how one-at-a-time mindsets are effective*. Routledge, forthcoming.

Rycroft, P., & Young, J. (2014). SST in Australia. In M.F. Hoyt & M. Talmon (Eds.), *Capturing moment: Single session therapy and walk-in services* (pp. 1410156). Crown House Publishing.

Rycroft, P., & Young, J. (2021). Translating single session thinking into practice. In M.F. Hoyt, J. Young, & P. Rycroft (Eds.), *Single session thinking and practice in global, cultural, and familial contexts* (pp. 42–53). Routledge.

Sagherian, M.J., Huedo-Medina, T.B., Pellowski, J.A., Eaton, L.A., & Johnson, B.T. (2016). Single-session behavioral interventions for sexual risk education: A meta-analysis. *Annals of Behavioral Medicine, 50*(6), 920–934.

Sahl, M. (1976). *Heartland*. Harcourt Brace Jovanovich.

Saladino, V. (Ed.) (2021). *Le strategic in psicoterapi.: Ricera e innovazione. [Strategies in psychotherapy: Research and innovations.]* Published in Italian. Cacucci Editore.

Santor, D.A., & Segal, Z.V. (2001). Predicting symptom return from rate of symptom reduction in cognitive-behavioral therapy for depression. *Cognitive Therapy and Research, 25,* 117–135.

Satir, V. (1988). *The new peoplemaking* (2nd ed.). Science and Behavior Books.

Scamardo, M., Bobele, M., & Biever, J.L. (2004). A new perspective on client dropouts. *Journal of Systemic Therapies, 23*(2), 27–38.

Schleider, J. (2024). *Little treatments, big effects: How to build meaningful moments that can transform your mental health.* Robinson.

Schleider, J.L., & Beidas, R.S. (2022, 23 September). Harnessing the Single-Session Intervention approach to promote scalable implementation of evidence-based practices in healthcare. *Frontiers in Health Services,* Section on Implementation Science, Vol. 2. https://doi.org/10.3389/frhs.2022.997406

Schleider, J.L., & Weisz, J.R. (2017). Little treatments, promising effects? Meta-analysis of single-session interventions for youth psychiatric problems. *Journal of the American Academy of Child and Adolescent Psychiatry, 56*(2), 107–115.

Schwartz, R.C. (2023). *Introduction to internal family systems.* Sounds Good Publications.

Sermijn, J., & Gergen, K. J. (2017). Spread the wings of your therapeutic potential: A reflecting process with Ken Gergen. *International Journal of Collaborative-Dialogic Practice, 8*(1), 57– 68.

Sharry, J., Madden B., & Darmody, M. (2001). *Becoming a solution detective: A strengths-based guide to brief therapy.* BT Press.

Sharry, J., Madden, B., Darmody, M., & Miller, S.D. (2001). Giving our clients the break: Applications of client-directed, outcome-informed clinical work. *Journal of Systemic Therapies, 20*(3), 68–76.

Shaver, B.J. (2009). *I'm gonna live forever.* Luck Films.

Shennan, G., & Iveson, C. (2012). From solution to description: Practice and research in tandem. In C. Franklin, T.S. Tepper, W.J. Gingerich, & E.E. McCollum (Eds.), *Solution-focused brief therapy: A handbook of evidence-based practice* (pp. 281–298). Oxford University Press.

Short, D.N (2021). What is Ericksonian therapy: The use of core competencies to operationally define a nonstandardized approach to psychotherapy. *Clinical Psychology: Science and Practice, 28*(3), 282–292.

Short, D.N. (2022). *Making psychotherapy more effective with unconscious process work.* Routledge.

Short, D.N., Erickson, B.A., & Klein, R.E. (2005). *Hope and resiliency: Understanding the psychotherapeutic strategies of Milton H. Erickson, M.D.* Crown House Publishing.

Silverman, W.H., & Beech, R.P. (1979). Are dropouts, dropouts? *Journal of Community Psychology, 7,* 236–242.

Simon, G.E., Imel, Z.E., Ludman, E.J., & Steinfield, B.J. (2012). Is dropout after the first psychotherapy visit always a bad thing? *Psychiatric Services, 63*(7), 705–707.

Singh, R. (1992). Single-session hypnotic treatment of insomnia in religious context. *Australian Journal of Clinical and Experimental Hypnosis, 20*(2), 111–116.

Singla, D.R., Schleider, J.L., & Patel, V. (2023). Democratizing access to psychological therapies: Innovations and the role of psychologists. *Journal of Consulting and Clinical Psychology, 91*(11), 623–625.

Slavin, J.H., & Rahmani, M. (2016). *Those 45 Minutes Changed My Life*: The meeting of Sigmund Freud and Margarethe Lutz. *Psychoanalytic Perspectives, 13*(3), 291–293. https://doi.org/10.1080/1551806X.2016.1228884

Slive, A., & Bobele, M. (Eds.) (2011). *When one hour is all you have: Effective therapy for walk-in clients.* Zeig, Tucker, & Theisen.

Slive, A., & Bobele, M. (2012). Walk-in counselling services: Making the most of one hour. *Australian and New Zealand Journal of Family Therapy, 33*(1), 27–38.

Slive, S., & Bobele, M. (2014). Walk-in single session therapy: Accessible mental health services. In M.F. Hoyt & M. Talmon (Eds.), *Capturing the moment: Single session therapy and walk-in services* (pp. 73–94). Crown House Publishing.

Slive, A., & Bobele, M. (2018). The three top reasons why walk-in/single-sessions make perfect sense. In M.F. Hoyt et al. (Eds.), *Single-session therapy by walk-in or appointment* (pp. 27–39). Routledge.

Slive, A., & Bobele, M. (2019a). Introduction to the special section: What's so scary about single-session therapy? *Journal of Systemic Therapies, 38*(4), 15–16.

Slive, A., & Bobele, M. (2019b). Ideas for addressing doubts about walk-in single-session therapy. *Journal of Systemic Therapies, 38*(4), 17–30.

Slive, A., & Bobele, M.B. (in press a). Open access single sessions: The SST model developed in Canada and Texas for walk-in, drop-in, and virtual services. In F. Cannistrà & M.F. Hoyt (Eds.), *Single session therapies: Why and how one-at-a-time mindsets are effective.* Routledge. Forthcoming.

Slive, A., & Bobele, M. (Eds.) (in press b). *Open access/one-at-a-time single session psychotherapy.* Routledge, forthcoming.

Slive, A., MacLaurin, B., Oaklander, M., & Amundson, J. (1995). Walk-in single sessions: A new paradigm in clinical service delivery. *Journal of Systemic Therapies, 14*, 3–11.

Slive, A., McElheran, N., & Lawson, A. (2008). How brief does it get? Walk-in single-session therapy. *Journal of Systemic Therapies, 27*(1), 5–22.

Sluzki, C.E. (1988). Case commentary II. *Family Therapy Networker, 12*(5), 77–81.

Sluzki, C.E. (1992). Transformations: A blueprint for narrative changes in therapy. *Family Process, 31*(3), 217–230.

Sluzki, C.E. (1998). Strange attractors and the transformation of narratives in family therapy. In M.F. Hoyt (Ed.), *The handbook of constructive therapies* (pp. 159–179). Jossey-Bass.

Snyder, C.R. (2002). Hope theory: Rainbows of the mind. *Psychological Inquiry, 13*(4), 249–275.

Söderquist, M. (2018). Coincidence favors the prepared mind: Single sessions with couples in Sweden. In M.F. Hoyt et al. (Eds.), *Single-session therapy by walk-in or appointment* (pp. 270–290). Routledge.

Söderquist, M. (2021). Making the leap with couples in Sweden: One-at-a-time mindset in action. In M.F. Hoyt, J. Young, & P. Rycroft (Eds.), *Single session thinking in global, cultural, and familial contexts* (pp. 163–172). Routledge.

Söderquist, M. (2023). *Single session one at a time counselling with couples: Challenge and possibility.* Routledge.

Söderquist, M., Cronholm-Nouicer, M., Dannerup, L., & Wulff, K. (2021). Making the leap with couples in Sweden: One-at-a-time mindset in action. In M.F. Hoyt, J. Young, & P. Rycroft (Eds.), *Single session thinking and practice in global, cultural, and familial contexts: Expanding applications* (pp. 163–172). Routledge.

Soo-Hoo, T. (2018). Working within the client's cultural context in single-session therapy. In M.F. Hoyt et al. (Eds.), *Single-session therapy by walk-in or appointment* (pp. 186–201). Routledge.

Sorensen, S. (2021). Hope in remote places: Single session therapy in Indigenous communities in Canada. In M.F. Hoyt, J. Young, & P. Rycroft (Eds.), *Single session thinking and practice in global, cultural, and familial contexts* (pp. 223–233). Routledge.

Sperry, L. (2010). Introduction: The art of being a failure as a therapist. In M. Richeport-Haley & J. Carlson (Eds.), *Jay Haley revisited* (pp. 73–91). Routledge.

Sperry, L., & Binensztok, V. (2019). *Ultra-brief cognitive behavioral interventions: A new practice model for mental health and integrated care*. Routledge.

Springmann, R.R. (1978). Single session psychotherapy in secondary male impotence. *Mental Health and Society, 5*, 86–93.

Sproel, O.H. (1975). Single-session psychotherapy. *Diseases of the Nervous System, 36*, 283–285.

Stadter, M. (1996). *Object relations brief therapy: The therapeutic relationship in short-term work*. Jason Aronson Publishers.

Stanton, H.E. (1991). Smoking cessation in a single session: An update. *International Journal of Psychosomatics, 38*(1–4), 84–88.

Steenbarger, B.N., (2002). Single-session therapy. In *Encyclopedia of psychology* (M. Hersen & W. Sledge, Eds.; Vol. 2, pp. 669–672). Academic Press.

Steenbarger, B.N. (2012). Solution-focused brief therapy: Doing what works. In M.J. Dewan, B.N. Steenbarger, & R.P. Greenberg (Eds.), *The art and science of brief psychotherapies: An illustrated guide* (2nd ed., pp. 121–155). American Psychiatric Publishing.

Stephenson, K. (2023, December). Single session thinking: Its global impact and role in therapeutic services. *Context, 190*, 29–31.

Stewart, J., McElheran, N., Park, H., Oakander, M., MacLaurin, B., Fang, C.J., & Robinson, A. (2018). Twenty-five years of walk-in single-sessions at the Eastside Family Centre; Clinical and research dimensions. In M.F. Hoyt et al. (Eds.), *Single-session therapy by walk-in or appointment* (pp. 72–90). Routledge.

Stiles, W.B., Leiman, M., Shapiro, D.A., Hardy, G.E., Barkham, M., Detert, N.B., & Llewelyn, S.P. (2006). What does the first exchange tell? Dialogical sequence analysis and assimilation in very brief therapy. *Psychotherapy Research, 16*(4), 408–421.

Stone, H. (2002). The thirty-minute counseling case. *Journal of Pastoral Counseling, 6*(1), 71–76.

Story, K. (2018). "Coming in for tune-ups": A family's experience of episodic long-term single- session therapy at the Bouverie Centre, Melbourne. In M.F. Hoyt et al. (Eds.), *Single- session therapy by walk-in or appointment* (pp. 202–220). Routledge.

Sue, D.W., & Sue, D. (2013). *Counseling the culturally diverse: Theory and practice* (6th ed.). Wiley.

Sullivan H.S. (1954). *The psychiatric interview*. Norton.

Swift, J.K., & Greenberg, R.P. (2012). Premature discontinuation in adult psychotherapy: A meta-analysis. *Journal of Consulting and Clinical Psychology, 80*(4), 547–559.

Taibbi, R. (2016). *The art of the first session: Making psychotherapy count from the start*. Norton.

Talmon, M. (1990). *Single-session therapy: Maximizing the effect of the first (and often only) therapeutic encounter*. Jossey-Bass.

Talmon, M. (1993). *Single session solutions: A guide to practical, effective, and affordable therapy*. Addison-Wesley.

Talmon, M. (2014). When less is more: Maximizing the effect of the first (and often only) therapeutic encounter. In M.F. Hoyt & M. Talmon (Eds.), *Capturing the moment: Single session therapy and walk-in services* (pp. 27–40). Crown House Publishing.

Talmon, M. (2018). The eternal now: On becoming and being a single-session therapist. In M.F. Hoyt et al. (Eds.), *Single-session therapy by walk-in or appointment* (pp. 149–154). Routledge.

Talmon, M. (2023, November 10). *The golden hour: SST as a life-long event.* Presentation at 4th International Symposium on Single Session Therapy, Rome.

Talmon, M., Hoyt, M.F., & Rosenbaum, R. (1990). Effective single-session therapy: Step-by- step guidelines. In M. Talmon (Ed.), *Single-session therapy: Maximizing the effect of the first (and often only) therapeutic encounter* (pp. 34–56). Jossey-Bass.

Talmon, M., Rosenbaum, R., Hoyt, M.F., & Short, L. (1990). *Single session therapy.* Videotape. Golden Triad Films.

Tilden, T., Solem, M.-B., Thuen, F., Lorås, L., Stokkebekk, J., & Whittaker, K. (2024). Taking empirical evidence seriously v.2.0. *Journal of Family Therapy*, early online. https://doi.org/10.1111/1467-6427.12448.

Tolchard, B., Thomas, L., & Battersby, M. (2006). Case reports and single session exposure therapy for problem gambling: A single-case experimental design. *Behavior Change*, *23*(2), 148–155.

Tolstoy, L. (1885). *What men live by, and other tales.* CreateSpace Independent Publishing Platform, 2016.

Tomm, K. (1992). *Interviewing the internalized other: Toward a systemic reconstruction of the self and other.* Workshop sponsored by the California School of Professional Psychology, Alameda, CA.

Tomm, K., Hoyt, M.F., & Madigan, S.P. (1998). Honoring our internalized others and the ethics of caring: A conversation with Karl Tomm. In M.F. Hoyt (Ed.), *The handbook of constructive therapies* (pp. 198–218). Jossey-Bass.

Torricelli, V. (2021). Single-session therapy: Cases. In F. Cannistrà & F. Piccirilli, *Single-session therapy: Principles and practices* (pp. 121–165). Giunti.

van der Veer, G. (2017). Training counsellors in low and middle income countries in single session counselling: Helping mental health and psychosocial workers to get on top of feelings of powerlessness. *Intervention, 15*(10), 70–75.

van Empel, H. (2023, November 12). Single Session Therapy in the corporate world. Invited address at 4th International Single Session Therapy Symposium, Rome.

van Empel, H. (in press). *Single Session Therapy: Help je Cliënt Korte en Krachtig Voorut [in Dutch] [Single Session Therapy: Help Your Client Move Forward Briefly and Powerfully].*

Vasconcelos, J.Q.M., & Neto, L.M. (2004) The "internalized other" interviewing technique revisited. *Journal of Family Psychotherapy, 14*(4), 15–26.

von Doussa, H., Tsorlinis, K., Cordukes, K., Beauchamp, J., & McIntosh, J.E. (2021). One-off sessions to address a waitlist: A pilot study. In M.F. Hoyt, J. Young, & P. Rycroft (Eds.), *Single session thinking and practice in global, cultural, and familial contexts* (pp. 117–124). Routledge.

Vitry, G., de Scorraille, C., & Hoyt, M.F. (2021). Redundant attempted solutions: 50 years of theory, evolution, and new supporting data. *Australian and New Zealand Journal of Family Therapy, 42*, 174–187.

Vitry, G., de Scorraille, C., Portelli, C., & Hoyt, M.F. (2021) Redundant attempted solutions: Operative diagnoses and strategic interventions to disrupt more of the same. *Journal of Systemic Therapies, 40*(4), 12–29.

Vitry, G., Pakrosnis, R., Jackson, J.B., Gallin, E., & Hoyt, M.F. (in press). Problem Resolution Scale (PRS): A single-item instrument for easily assessing clinical improvement. *Journal of Marital and Family Therapy*, forthcoming.

von Glaserfeld, E. (1995). *Radical constructivism: A way of knowing and learning.* The Palmer Press.

Walter, J.L., & Peller, J.E. (1994). "On track" in solution-focused brief therapy. In M.F. Hoyt (Ed.), *Constructive therapies* (pp. 111–125). Guilford Press.

Walton, G.M., & Cohen, G.L. (2011). A brief social-belonging intervention improves academic and health outcomes of minority students. *Science, 331,* 1447–1451.

Watzlawick, P. (1978). *The language of change: Elements of therapeutic communication.* Norton.

Watzlawick, P. (Ed.) (1984). *The invented reality: How do we know what we believe we know? (Contributions to constructivism).* Norton.

Watzlawick, P., Beavin, J.B., & Jackson, D.D. (1967). *Pragmatics of human communication: A study of interactional patterns, pathologies, and paradoxes.* Norton.

Watzlawick, P., Weakland, J.H., & Fisch, R. (1974). *Change: Principles of problem formation and problem resolution.* Norton.

Weakland, J.H. (1988). Weakland on the Woodys-Bobele exchange. *Journal of Marital ad Family Therapy, 14*(2), 205.

Weakland, J.H., & Fisch, R. (1992). Brief therapy – MRI style. In S.H. Budman, M.F. Hoyt, & S. Friedman (Eds.), *The first session in brief therapy* (pp. 306–323). Guilford Press.

Weeks, G.R., & L. L'Abate (1982). *Paradoxical psychotherapy: Theory and practice with individuals, couples, and families.* Routledge.

Weiner-Davis, M. (1992). *Divorce busting: A step-by-step approach to making your marriage loving again.* Simon & Schuster.

Weiner-Davis, M. (1993). Pro-constructed realities. In S. Gilligan & R. Price (Eds.), *Therapeutic conversations* (pp. 149–157). Norton.

Weiner-Davis, M., de Shazer, S., & Gingrich, W.J. (1987). Using pretreatment change to construct a therapeutic solution: An exploratory study. *Journal of Marital and Family Therapy, 13,* 359–363.

Weir, S., Wills, M., Young, J., & Perlesz, A. (2008). *The implementation of single session work in community health.* The Bouverie Centre, La Trobe University (Australia).

Wells, J. E., Browne, M. O., Aguilar-Gaxiola, S., Al-Hamzawi, A., Alonso, J., Angermeyer, M. C., ... & Kessler, R. C. (2013). Drop out from out-patient mental healthcare in the World Health organization's World mental Health Survey initiative. *British Journal of Psychiatry, 202*(1), 42–49.

Wender, P. (1968). Vicious and virtuous circles: The role of deviation amplifying feedback in the origin and perpetuation of behavior. *Psychiatry, 31,* 309–324.

Westmacott, R., & Hunsley, J. (2010) Reasons for terminating psychotherapy: A general population study. *Journal of Clinical Psychology, 66*(9), 965–977.

Westwater, J.J., Murphy, M., Handley, C., & McGregor, L. (2020). A mixed methods exploration of single session family therapy in a child and adolescent mental health service in Tasmania, Australia. *Australian and New Zealand Journal of Family Therapy, 41,* 258–270 https://doi.org/10.1002/anzf.1420

Whitaker, C.A. (1975). Psychotherapy of the absurd: With a special emphasis on the psychotherapy of aggression. *Family Process, 4,* 1–16.

Whitaker, C.A. (1976). The hindrance of theory in clinical work. In P.J. Guerin (Ed.), *Family therapy: Theory and practice* (pp. 154–164). Gardner Press. Reprinted in J.R. Neill

& D.P. Kniskern (Eds.), *From psyche to system: The evolving therapy of Carl Whitaker* (pp. 317–329). Guilford Press, 1982.

Whitaker, C.A. (1983). Comment. *Voices, 19,* 40.

Whitaker, C.A. (1990, December). *Symbolic experiential family therapy: Model and methodology.* Paper presented at The Evolution of Psychotherapy: A Conference. Anaheim, CA. A version in J.K. Zeig (Ed.), *The evolution of psychotherapy: The second conference* (pp. 13–20). Brunner/Mazel.

White, M. (1989). Saying hullo again: The incorporation of the lost relationship in the resolution of grief. In *Selected papers* (pp. 29–36). Dulwich Centre Publications.

White, M. (1992). Family therapy training and supervision in a world of experience and narrative. In D. Epston & M. White (Eds.), *Experience, contradiction, narrative & imagination: Selected papers of David Epston & Michael White 1989–1991* (pp. 75–95). Dulwich Centre Publications.

White, M. (1997). *Narratives of therapists' lives.* Dulwich Centre Publications.

White, M. (2007). *Maps of narrative practice.* Norton.

White, M., & Epston, D. (1990). *Narrative means to therapeutic ends.* Norton.

Whitman, W. (1940). Song of myself. In *Leaves of grass* (J. Kouwenhoven, Editor; rev. ed., pp. 29–74). Modern Library/Random House. (work originally published 1881–1882)

Wilkerson, I. (2020). *Caste: The origins of our discontents.* Random House.

Williams, J.M., & Hall, D.W. (1988). Use of single session hypnosis for smoking cessation. *Addictive Behaviors, 13*(2), 205–208.

Winnicott, D.W. (1949). Hate in the countertransference. *International Journal of Psychoanalysis, 30,* 69–74.

Winnicott, D.W. (1958). *Through paediatrics to psychoanalysis.* Basic Books.

Winnicott, D.W. (1986). *Home is where we start from: Essays by a psychoanalyst.* Norton.

Wolberg, L.R. (1965). The technic of short-term psychotherapy. In L.R. Wolberg (Ed.), *Short- term psychotherapy* (pp. 127–200). Grune & Stratton.

Wolberg, L.R. (1980). Catalyzing the therapeutic process: The use of hypnosis. In L.R. Wolberg (Ed.), *Handbook of short-term psychotherapy.* Grune & Stratton.

Wolpe, J. (1958). *Psychotherapy by reciprocal inhibition.* Stanford University Press.

Yalom, I., & Leszcz, M. (2005). *The theory and practice of group psychotherapy* (5th ed.). Basic Books.

Yapko, M.D. (1989). Disturbances of temporal orientation as a feature of depression. In M.D. Yapko (Ed.), *Brief therapy approaches to treating anxiety and depression* (pp. 106–118). Brunner/Mazel.

Yapko, M.D. (1990a). The case of Vicki: Hypnosis for coping with terminal cancer. In M.D. Yapko, *Trancework* (2nd ed., pp. 347–404). Brunner/Mazel.

Yapko, M.D. (1990b). Brief therapy tactics in longer-term psychotherapies. In J.K. Zeig & S.G. Gilligan (Eds.), *Brief therapy: Myths, methods, and metaphors* (pp. 185–195). Brunner/Mazel.

Yapko, M.D. (2012). *Trancework: An introduction to the practice of clinical hypnosis* (4th ed.). Routledge.

Young, J. (2018). Single-session therapy: The misunderstood gift that keeps on giving. In M.F. Hoyt et al. (Eds.), *Single-session therapy by walk-in or appointment* (pp. 40–58). Routledge.

Young, J. (2024). *No bullshit therapy: How to engage people who don't want to work with you.* Routledge.

Young, J., & Rycroft, P. (1997). Single session therapy: Capturing the moment. *Psychotherapy in Australia, 4*(10), 18–23.

Young, J., Rycroft, P., & Weir, S. (2014). Implementing single session therapy: Practical wisdoms from Down Under. In M.F. Hoyt & M. Talmon (Eds.), *Capturing the moment* (pp. 121–140). Crown House Publishing.

Young, K. (2011a). When all the time you have is now: Re-visiting practices and narrative therapy in a walk-in clinic. In J. Duvall & L. Beres (Eds.), *Innovations in narrative therapy: Connecting practice, training, and research* (pp. 147–166). Norton.

Young, K. (2011b). Narrative practices at a walk-in therapy clinic. In A. Slive & M. Bobele (Eds.), *When one hour is all you have: Effective therapy for walk-in clients* (pp. 149–166). Zeig, Tucker, & Theisen.

Young, K. (2017). Walk-in therapy clinics: An opportunity for socially just conversations. In D.A. Paré & C. Audet (Eds.), *Social justice and counselling: Discourse in practice* (pp. 212–224). Routledge.

Young, K. (2018). Change in the winds: The growth of walk-in therapy clinics in Ontario, Canada. In M.F. Hoyt et al. (Eds.), *Single-session therapy by walk-in or appointment* (pp. 59–71). Routledge.

Young, K., & Bhanot-Malhotra, S. (2014). *Getting services right: An Ontario multi-agency evaluation study.* www.windzcentre.com

Young, K., & Jebreen, J. (2020). Recognizing single-session therapy as psychotherapy. *Journal of Systemic Therapies, 38*(4), 31–44.

Zeig, J.K. (Ed.) (1980). *A teaching seminar with Milton H. Erickson, M.D.* Brunner/Mazel.

Zeig, J.K. (2018). *The anatomy of experiential impact through Ericksonian psychotherapy: Seeing, doing, being.* Milton H. Erickson Foundation Press.

Zeig, J.K. (2022a). *An epic life: Milton H. Erickson professional perspectives.* The Milton H. Erickson Foundation.

Zeig, J. (2022b). *An epic life II: Milton H. Erickson personal perspectives.* The Milton H. Erickson Foundation Press.

Zeigarnik, B. (1938). On finished and unfinished tasks. In W.D. Ellis (Ed.), *A source book of Gestalt psychology.* Harcourt Brace Jovanovich. Summarized in J.W. Atkinson, *An introduction to motivation.* Van Nostrand Reinhold, 1964.

Ziadni, M.S., Chen, A.L., Winslow, T., Mackey, S.C., & Darnell, B.D. (2020). Efficacy and mechanisms of a single-session behavioral medicine class among patients with chronic pain taking prescription opioids: Study protocol for a randomized controlled trial. *BMC Trials, 21,* 521.

Ziadni, M.S., Gonzalez-Castro, L., Anderson, S., Krishnamurthy, P., & Darnall, B.D. (2021). Efficacy of a single-session "empowered relief" Zoom-delivered group intervention for chronic pain: Randomized controlled trial conducted during the COVID-19 pandemic. *Journal of Medical Internet Research, 23*(9), e29672. https://doi.org/10.2196/29672

Ziegler, P.B., & Hiller, T. (2001). *Recreating partnership: A solution-oriented, collaborative approach to couples therapy.* Norton.

Ziegler, P.B., & Hoyt, M.F. (2023, September). Effective goal-constructing conversation in single session/brief therapy. *The Science of Psychotherapy, 11*(9), 20–29 (online).

Zirkle, G. (1961). Five-minute psychotherapy. *American Journal of Psychiatry, 118,* 544–546.

Index

Note: *Italic* page numbers refer to figures and page numbers followed by "n" denote footnotes.

Printed in the United States
by Baker & Taylor Publisher Services